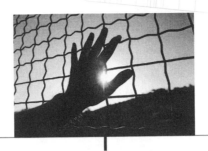

THE **PSYCHIATRIC EVALUATION**
AND
TREATMENT OF REFUGEES

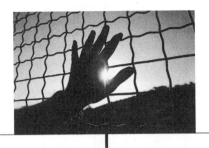

THE **PSYCHIATRIC EVALUATION**
AND
TREATMENT OF REFUGEES

Edited by

J. David Kinzie, M.D.

George A. Keepers, M.D.

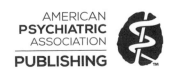

AMERICAN
PSYCHIATRIC
ASSOCIATION
PUBLISHING

Copyright © 2020 American Psychiatric Association Publishing

ALL RIGHTS RESERVED

First Edition

Manufactured in the United States of America on acid-free paper
24 23 22 21 20   5 4 3 2 1

American Psychiatric Association Publishing
800 Maine Avenue SW
Suite 900
Washington, DC 20024-2812
www.appi.org

Library of Congress Cataloging-in-Publication Data
Names: Kinzie, J. David, editor. | Keepers, George A., editor. | American Psychiatric Association Publishing, issuing body.
Title: The psychiatric evaluation and treatment of refugees / edited by J. David Kinzie, George A. Keepers.
Description: First edition. | Washington, DC : American Psychiatric Association Publishing, [2020] | Includes bibliographical references and index.
Identifiers: LCCN 2020007082 | ISBN 9781615372263 (paperback) | ISBN 9781615373093 (ebook)
Subjects: MESH: Refugees—psychology | Mental Disorders—diagnosis | Interview, Psychological—methods | Culturally Competent Care | Emigrants and Immigrants—psychology | Psychological Trauma
Classification: LCC RC451.4.R43 | NLM WA 305.1 | DDC 616.890086/912—dc23
LC record available at https://lccn.loc.gov/2020007082

British Library Cataloguing in Publication Data
A CIP record is available from the British Library

Contents

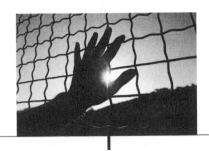

CONTRIBUTORS

Erike Apolinar, LMFT
Director of Psychotherapy Services, Sun Valley Behavioral and Research Centers, Imperial, California

James Boehnlein, M.D.
Professor, Department of Psychiatry, Oregon Health & Science University, Portland, Oregon

Keith Cheng, M.D.
Clinical Associate Professor, Division of Child Psychiatry, Oregon Health & Science University, Portland, Oregon

James Griffith, M.D.
Leon M. Yochelson Professor and Chair, Department of Psychiatry and Behavioral Sciences, George Washington University, Washington, D.C.

George A. Keepers, M.D., FACPsych, DLFAPA
Carruthers Professor and Chair, Department of Psychiatry, Oregon Health & Science University, Portland, Oregon

J. David Kinzie, M.D., FACPsych, DLFAPA
Professor, Department of Psychiatry, Oregon Health & Science University, Portland, Oregon

Mark Kinzie, M.D., Ph.D.
Associate Professor, Department of Psychiatry, Oregon Health & Science University, Portland, Oregon

Paul Leung, M.D.
Clinical Professor, Department of Psychiatry, Oregon Health & Science University, Portland, Oregon

Mario A. Martinez, M.D.
Chief of Children and Adolescent Outpatient Services, Instituto Psiquiátrico del Estado de Baja California, Mexicali, Baja California, Mexico

Bernardo Ng, M.D., FAPA
Medical Director, Sun Valley Behavioral and Research Centers, Imperial, California

Linda Piwowarczyk, M.D., M.P.H.
Boston Center for Refugee Health & Human Rights, Boston Medical Center; Assistant Professor in Psychiatry, Boston University School of Medicine, Boston, Massachusetts

Daryn Reicherter, M.D.
Clinical Professor, Department of Psychiatry and Behavioral Sciences, Stanford University

Derrick Silove, A.M., M.B. Ch.B. (Hons I), M.D., FRANZCP, FASSA
Scientia Professor, School of Psychiatry, University of New South Wales, Kensington, Sydney, Australia

Sara Teichholtz, M.D.
Resident, Department of Psychiatry and Behavioral Sciences, George Washington University, Washington, D.C.

Dhanviney Verma, M.D.
Instructor in Psychiatry, Harvard Medical School, Massachusetts General Hospital, Boston, Massachusetts

Ronald Wintrob, M.D.
Past President, Society for the Study of Psychiatry and Culture

Paria Zarrinnegar, M.D.
Postdoctoral Fellow, Division of Child Psychiatry, Oregon Health & Science University, Portland, Oregon

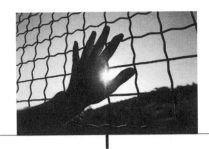

ACKNOWLEDGMENTS

The authors appreciate the excellent logistical support from Desiree Batiste and Samantha Birk and the fine editorial corrections and additions from Crystal Riley, M.A.

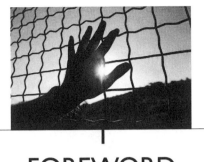

FOREWORD

Throughout its history, America has seen itself, and been seen by other nations, as a country open to and welcoming of immigrants, as symbolized by the Statue of Liberty in New York Harbor. The degree to which public sentiment and government policies have been supportive toward immigrants, refugees, and asylum seekers has fluctuated from enthusiastic welcome for those who were fleeing from discrimination, persecution, poverty, and natural disasters in their home countries, to fear and antipathy toward immigrants from specific ethnic, racial, and religious backgrounds.

Immigration numbers peaked in America in the first decades of the twentieth century, then sharply decreased from 15% of the total U.S. population in the 1920s to 5% in the 1970s, reflecting changes in public support and government policy toward immigrants. By the first decade of the twenty-first century, the proportion of immigrants in the U.S. population had once again reached 15% of the total U.S. population—equivalent to what it had been in the first decade of the twentieth century.

In recent years, fear of terrorism has merged with fear of immigrants—and especially fear of refugees and asylum seekers from countries in Asia, Africa, and Latin America suffering from protracted internal conflict, war, drought, food shortages, and both political and economic instability. These developments have been increasingly evident in Europe as well as in America, resulting in sharply increased public hostility and governmental policy restrictions—not only toward immigrants but also, in particular, toward refugees and asylum seekers viewed as a burden and as a threat to the social, cultural, economic, and political stability of the nation.

It is this context that gives even greater strength and validity to the chapters in this volume, edited by J. David Kinzie and George A. Keepers, devoted to the best practices in psychiatric assessment and treatment of refugees and drawn from the experience of the Intercultural Psychiatric Program (IPP) at the Oregon Health & Science University (OHSU) in Portland, Oregon. In existence for over 40 years, the IPP has established and maintained a clinical service for refugees and asylum seekers who have come to America seeking safety, liberty, acceptance, and opportunity during those years.

In his clearly written overview of cultural and diagnostic issues in refugees, James Boehnlein cites the 2018 report of the United Nations High Commissioner for Refugees (UNHCR) indicating that there are 66 million forcibly displaced people in the world, of whom 22 million are refugees, who are unable to return to their country of origin based on their well-founded fear of persecution due to race, religion, nationality, political opinions, or membership in a specific social group.

Since 2000, approximately 75,000 migrants have entered the United States each year as refugees. The numbers authorized in 2015 and 2016 were increased to 110,000 per year, specifically to accommodate the surge of migrants from war-torn Iraq, Syria, and Afghanistan. However, in fiscal year 2016, reflecting a government policy change marked by increasing intolerance of refugees and asylum seekers from those countries, the number of refugees admitted to the United States was less than 85,000. In 2017, that number decreased again, to 54,000, with the approval ceiling for 2018 being lower still.

Boehnlein notes that despite the conditions of persecution, deprivation, physical danger, loss of physical and financial security, and separation from and loss of family, as well as fear of and experience of abuse and violence in refugee camps prior to resettlement in United States, there currently is no clear evidence that prevalence rates of mental disorders among refugees in the initial years of resettlement are significantly higher or lower than those in the host population, with the exception of psychosis and PTSD. However, over the long term, among resettled refugees, the rates of depression and anxiety disorders seem to be higher, and rates of PTSD remain at a higher level than in the host population. Ongoing separation from family members in the country of origin has been found to be a significant risk factor for poor refugee mental health postresettlement.

In their chapter on refugee children and families, Keith Cheng and
Paria Zarrinnegar cite the 2017 UNHCR report indicating that worldwide, there are approximately 10 million refugee children below the age
of 18. They also point to the recent changes in American public attitudes and government policy toward immigrants and refugees that have
resulted in uncoordinated—and increasingly protracted—discriminatory
and deleterious treatment of refugee children and families assigned to detention centers in some southern U.S. border facilities. They emphasize
that these conditions of detention and protracted screening can traumatize children, with results that are as devastating as those of armed political conflict and displacement to refugee camps prior to resettlement
in the United States. The authors point to recent policy changes intended
to discourage refugees seeking asylum in the United States by separating
refugee children from their accompanying parents and/or other family
members, and deporting parents without their children, as well as holding
unaccompanied youth and even young children in facilities unequipped to
handle the physical and psychological needs of such children and youth,
thereby increasing their risk of long-term developmental trauma. They
address the complex issue of acculturative stress for immigrant, refugee,
and asylum-seeking children, youth, and families in the face of negative
stereotyping, economic and educational disadvantage, and acculturative
stress—referring to concepts of vertical and horizontal identity formation, as developed by the psychologist Andrew Solomon in his 2013 book
Far From the Tree. Solomon relates vertical identity formation to attitudes
and values held by parents, reflecting their cultural upbringing and intended to be passed on to their children, whereas horizontal identity is
derived from children's exposure to peers and the youth culture of the postmigration host community, a frequent context of intrafamilial acculturative stress in immigrant families.

In his chapter outlining the IPP at OHSU and its treatment model
for refugees, David Kinzie describes a number of features characteristic
of refugees, including experience of forced migration from their homeland and multiple episodes of abusive and traumatic treatment prior to,
during, and postmigration—including death of family members, personal
torture, starvation, and prolonged time spent living in unsafe refugee
camps. In America, refugees are easily overwhelmed by the bureaucratic
procedures they encounter trying to arrange for housing, medical care,
and education for their children, and they are also stressed by the lack of a
secure income—in addition to poor adaptation to the host culture, ghet-
toization, and often xenophobic reactions from the host community.
Those who suffer from mental illness are even further disadvantaged by

fear of family and community rejection, an inability to make decisions, and stigma. More recently, there is an additional and very real threat of arbitrary detention and deportation by immigration authorities.

For a psychiatric program to be successful, it must accommodate the language of refugees, show respect for their cultural traditions and behaviors, understand the traumas and tragedies of their life experience, and above all have empathy for refugees. Patients are treated by a team that includes a psychiatrist, as well as a counselor who is a member of their ethnic group. Most counselors have master's degrees in counseling. Kinzie describes the counselors as "the glue that holds the patient and the program together." Research has been another fundamental component of the IPP, leading to publication of over 100 academic articles and book chapters to date.

Details of the psychiatric assessment and the treatement—both biological and psychological—of refugee individuals and families are described in the overview chapter and subsequent chapters focusing on children, youth and families, adult patients, and elderly refugees (including the impact of dementia on patients and the ethos of families caring for their elderly members without recourse to outside help). Approaches to adapting individual, group, and family psychotherapy, including specific techniques involved, are addressed. Each chapter includes illustrative clinical case examples of diverse issues in assessment and treatment.

Several authors emphasize that working with refugees and survivors of torture is often a long-standing process that requires developing patient-physician bonds that transcend time. Grasping the emotional impact of refugees' displacement from their homeland, family, community, and cultural traditions, in addition to confronting and coping with the categorical hatred, abuse, and violence faced by refugees in their home countries due to their ethnic and/or religious identity, requires a moral sensibility in therapists that extends beyond cultural competence. The emotional consequences of categorical hatred extend beyond symptoms of depression or PTSD. A fractured sense of identity, loss of a capacity to trust others, self-loathing, and loss of empathy for one's own suffering can be other consequences. Individuals often suffer shame from internalized stigmatization.

It can be a profoundly humbling experience for treatment personnel to accompany patients through their process of recovery—to be witnesses to both the worst of humanity and the strength and resilience of the human spirit. The work can be very challenging, and therapists do feel overwhelmed at times by the extent of the losses and suffering their patients have had to endure. However, to see such people recover their self-esteem and be able, once again, to show trust and resilience during their recovery, and to establish independently functioning lives in their resettlement communities, inspires therapists to embrace and continue this work. Providing care for refugees and asylum seekers is a complex but gratifying experience for a psychiatrist. It can expand a psychiatrist's repertoire of clinical skills through its focus on assessment and care for normal syndromes of distress, ethnopharmacology, family-centered care, and human rights advocacy. It encourages the development of a resilience-building approach to treatment. Providing care for a refugee becomes an opportunity not only to treat symptoms of illness but to help the person who has been disinherited regain his or her humanity—and as a result of that process, helps to validate and maintain the humanitarian instincts and integrity of therapists.

The psychiatric assessment and treatment of traumatized refugees raises a wide range of ethical issues. These issues are thoughtfully addressed in the chapter by Derrick Silove, based on the clinical and research activities of Silove and colleagues at the University of New South Wales in Sydney, Australia, over the past two decades. Silove points out that the nature of the refugee experience invariably results in a blurring between the considerations of clinical ethics, which focuses primarily on the doctor-patient relationship, and the broader human rights domain that extends to the relationship of the individual and group to the state, especially in the case of prolonged detention of asylum seekers in facilities closed to public scrutiny and intended, as government policy, to discourage and deter immigration. Under these emotionally and politically charged circumstances, currently evident in America and Europe as well as in Australia, the term *refugee* itself can be used in a pejorative and discriminatory manner, especially if it is affixed to the person as a permanent label—a process of reification that psychiatrists and other mental health professionals should actively discourage.

Increasingly, Silove notes, refugees and asylum seekers are being confined for indefinite periods to detention centers in prisonlike conditions, although they have not committed any crime. These facilities can be described as regimented environments that lack schooling and play facilities for children and have inadequate medical and psychiatric services. They have also been shown to expose these refugees and asylum seekers to risk of neglect, abuse, and violence, as well as confrontations with supervisory staff who lack significant training or clinical experience with physically and/or mentally ill refugees. Prolonged detention can retraumatize these people, exacerbating preestablished traumatic stress disorders. Detained asylum seekers, including children, exhibit unusually high rates of PTSD, depression, and anxiety; the stressors and traumas experienced in detention play a major role in perpetuating these symptoms, and psychiatric disturbances tend to persist in detainees for years. The tendency to label refugees and asylum seekers as illegal immigrants to justify harsh policies aimed at deterring their immigration and postmigration resettlement runs counter to the principles of international covenants such as the Universal Declaration of Human Rights and the United Nations Convention Related to the Status of Refugees, which clearly state that seeking asylum as a refuge from persecution is a right, not a crime.

Reflecting on the current unwelcoming public attitude and the negative stereotyping of refugees and asylum seekers in America and many other countries that have been the main providers of refuge and postmigration integration of immigrants for generations, and in light of the increasing hostility toward immigrants as government policy in those countries, Kinzie and Keepers lament these changes and their deleterious impact on all immigrants. They especially identify the rejection of asylum seekers; the overt prejudice toward asylum seekers from Asian, African, and Latin American countries; the specific refusal to accept asylum applicants from "Muslim countries"; and the facile characterization of immigrants as criminals and/or terrorists. They note the negative consequences of these attitudes on the human dignity, security, self-esteem, and overall stress among all categories of immigrants, not just refugees and asylum seekers. The negative implications for the mental health and cultural integration of all immigrants are clear. The various authors of this book lament the attendant rise of hate speech, of bigotry, and of overt racial, ethnic, and religious discrimination in American society. Such changes undermine the idealism and humanitarian instincts of all those who want to provide care and treatment of immigrants and are dedicated to the humanitarian ideals of cultural diversity, integration, and tolerance.

Ronald Wintrob, M.D.
Past President, Society for the Study of Psychiatry and Culture

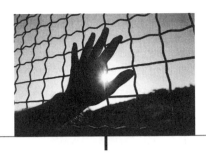

PREFACE

Unless the water is safer . . .

I walked along a serene, rocky Greek beach after a day spent in the refugee camps meeting survivors and learning about the arduous road they traveled. The deep blue Aegean Sea quelled the blazing sun. Many of the refugees had been subjected to human rights violations. The trauma had clearly affected their minds. As a trauma psychiatrist, my role for those in the camp was to describe the mental health outcomes of their traumas. The refugee camp was filled with persons who had come from different situations, spoke different languages, and had different cultures. There are many common mental outcomes of trauma, similar despite the diversity.

I walked along the beach to clear my mind.

The islands of Greece have become a repository for waves of refugees seeking sanctuary from war, torture, and persecution from Syria, Afghanistan, and Iran. They have endured more trauma than many can imagine. In the camps in the European Union, their hopes and their dreams for a future of freedom are on hold.

Medical science has amassed a great body of knowledge in regard to trauma's effect on mental health. There is an updated brain science of trauma, genetic science of trauma, clinical science of trauma, and population science of trauma. Psychiatrists have an art of how to contribute to the solutions for these effects. Clinical wisdom has led to an evidence base for the proactive field of trauma psychiatry. *Psychiatric Evaluation and Treatment of Refugees* is a cutting-edge volume of contributions that help mental health professionals better understand the outcomes and the solutions for the complicated mix of trauma and immigration with culture and worldview. Written by experts in cross-cultural psychiatry, the book holds a balance between the up-to-date science and the collective experiential wisdom of the Intercultural Psychiatric Program at the Oregon Health & Science University (OHSU). The authors have become key references for psychiatrists working in cross-cultural trauma for decades.

The authors' ideas are foundational to how I approach cross-cultural trauma psychiatry. Their science has been in my head throughout the moments I have been in contact with Greek camps.

When one has seen enough detention centers, refugee camps, and holding areas crammed with people, these camps begin to look the same. They are unimpressive. The people's destitute predicament draws compassion. The most remarkable aspect is always the humanity that the survivors bring to refugee camps. They adapt and personalize the deplorable conditions. They create humanity in places that otherwise would have none. But so often the traumatic experiences have taken a toll on their mental health and intervention is needed.

Their psychology is affected. They suffer. And they remember suffering. The memory of suffering is their past and their present.

If we think only in terms of diagnostic naming or in terms of statistics, the survivors become faceless numbers behind fences and barbed wire. Consideration of the science of trauma psychology in the context of real humanity is necessary to be effective in creating positive change. The editors and authors of this volume have contributed to our understanding of the blend of necessary science/evidence with compassion that gives mental health providers insight as to how to understand and treat. How else do we propose to treat without a science? How could we move forward without an evidence base? How would we practice without a guideline to the human art? This book suggests answers to these practical questions during a time when immigration is a global health concern and refugee populations are mounting. Traumatization among refugees is not a local concern; it is among the most challenging global health situations in modern times.

I continued walking along the beach. It was hot. I could not get my head straight for all the stories of flight spinning in my imagination. The sea was beautiful to look at but difficult to think about, as it is the carrier of refugee traffic by raft. And it swallows the same victims without any conscience. Yesterday's local newspaper told the story of a woman who drowned during her family's crossing—leaving an infant and a toddler motherless. Who will help her orphaned children? I kept walking along the beach. I could see the mainland on the horizon. The persecution happens there, and the camps are here. Between persecution and freedom is the sea—filled sometimes with hope, sometimes with despair, and often with death.

As Warsan Shire, a survivor/advocate, writes in her poem "Home,"

> you have to understand,
> that no one puts their children in a boat
> unless the water is safer than the land
> no one burns their palms
> under trains
> beneath carriages
> no one spends days and nights in the stomach of a truck
> feeding on newspaper unless the miles travelled
> means something more than journey

Imagine the state of a family's destitution when they have come to the point where "water is safer than the land." And they must engage danger and place their children in danger in order to escape. The land was their home. Now it has become unsafe. "No one leaves home until home is a sweaty voice in your ear / saying— /leave, / run away from me now / i dont know what I've become."

I looked down at the smoothed stones that clacked together in the delicate waves. One stone was so white against the others that it insisted closer inspection. But as I examined closer, I realized that it was no stone at all. It was the polished head of a human arm bone. No mistake. Smoothed by the sea, this one fragment had been polished for a long time. The bone presumably belonged to a person who must have made the long journey and endured much, only to end in tragedy.

For the victims there is death. For the survivors there is hope. But their psychology will be forever affected.

I am grateful for the academic contributions of Drs. David Kinzie and George Keepers, and their colleagues at the OHSU. I have, for decades, been the beneficiary of their clarification of this knowledge. Their scientific additions have aided and shaped the understanding of trauma psychology in refugees and immigrants. And, their compassionate approach to patient care has created clinical wisdom that all in the field can benefit from. I am honored to call them colleagues. This book, *The Psychiatric Evaluation and Treatment of Refugees*, is a necessary tool for the understanding of human trauma psychology and a guide for the well-being of the survivors. This volume appears during a time when guidance toward the psychological and physical recovery of traumatized refugees is essential. This book is a key to unlock the hope of the persons who have crossed the sea. And it is the key to ensure that the refugees have found land that is safer than water.

Daryn Reicherter, M.D.
Clinical Professor, Department of Psychiatry and Behavioral Sciences, Stanford University

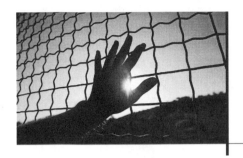

Chapter 1

OVERVIEW OF CULTURAL AND DIAGNOSTIC ISSUES

James Boehnlein, M.D.

Migration has been a part of the human condition since the beginning of time. People have traveled from one part of the world to another for a number of reasons. Some were looking for a better life, others wanted to see what was around the next corner, and many people over thousands of years have left their original places of habitation to escape adversity. This did not change in the twentieth century and continues in the twenty-first century. Unfortunately, conditions in various parts of the world have created difficult conditions for individuals, families, and communities because of war, persecution, or natural disasters. There are millions of migrants displaced not only within their own countries but also in various parts of the world. There currently are 66 million forcibly displaced people, of whom 22 million are refugees, more than half from Syria, Afghanistan, and South Sudan (United Nations High Commissioner for Refugees 2019). Refugees are a specific category of migrants: they are persons who are outside of their country of origin who are unable to return

1

to that country because of a well-founded fear of persecution due to race, religion, nationality, political opinions, or membership in a specific social group (United Nations High Commissioner for Refugees 2019). Asylum seekers are different from refugees as a group; asylum seekers apply for protection after they arrive in the country in which they are seeking safety rather than being screened and approved for refugee status as refugees are. Those applications can be in refugee camps or at designated sites outside their home countries (Refugee Health Technical Assistance Center 2011).

In this chapter, I begin by describing briefly the process by which refugees are screened for resettlement in the United States. I include recent data regarding countries of origin and describe some of the conditions in those countries of origin that give rise to refugee migration. I then discuss the challenges that refugees face prior to migration, during migration, and after arrival in the host country. In addition, I provide an overview of basic medical and psychiatric screening of refugees in mental health settings and briefly describe the various approaches to treatment that are discussed in more detail in other chapters in this book.

OVERVIEW OF RESETTLEMENT: SCREENING AND DEMOGRAPHICS

THE REFUGEE SCREENING PROCESS

The United States is a party of the 1967 United Nations Protocol Relating to the Status of Refugees that incorporated articles of the original 1951 Refugee Convention (United Nations High Commission for Refugees 2011). Because the United States is a signatory of the United Nations protocol, it is obligated to protect refugees seeking asylum from persecution. Congress legislated U.S. obligations under the United States protocol when it codified refugee protection and the procedures for asylum in the Refugee Act of 1980 (Administration for Children and Families 2012). After fleeing their own country, refugees most commonly stop at refugee camps on the border of their country or in camps in neighboring countries. If they wish to be resettled, refugees are screened by the United Nations High Commissioner for Refugees (UNHCR) to determine whether they are eligible for refugee status and qualify for UNHCR protection. The process of resettlement can often be very lengthy.

The first step in being resettled in the United States is an interview with an officer of the U.S. Citizenship and Immigration Services to determine eligibility and to arrange a required medical examination and security clearances (Refugee Health Technical Assistance Center 2011). The medical examination that occurs overseas before the refugee is accepted for resettlement in the United States screens for communicable diseases that have an impact on public health such as tuberculosis, syphilis and other sexually transmitted diseases, and leprosy. In addition, applicants are screened for drug addiction and any condition that would create conditions for harmful behaviors. If a refugee passes medical screening and security clearance overseas, he or she is granted refugee status by the U.S. Department of Homeland Security and is brought to the United States for resettlement by the U.S. Department of State. Voluntary agencies and the U.S. Department of Health and Human Services's U.S. Office of Refugee Resettlement assist with resettlement in the United States (Administration for Children and Families 2019).

Once refugees arrive in the United States, the U.S. Department of State has cooperative agreements with resettlement agencies to provide services for refugees. The Office of Refugee Settlement is the lead agency for domestic refugee programs. These services include food, clothing, housing, employment, and medical care during the first 90 days after arrival. In reality, most refugee resettlement agencies provide longer-term support for refugees after arrival in the United States. Most refugees are also eligible for 8 months of short-term health insurance called Refugee Medical Assistance (Administration for Children and Families 2019), and the Affordable Care Act permits refugees to be eligible for medical care in states that provide funding through the marketplace exchanges.

COUNTRIES OF ORIGIN

Since the end of the Vietnam War in 1975, refugees have come to the United States from a variety of regions. From the mid-1970s through the 1980s, the vast majority of refugees settling in the United States came from Southeast Asia. The largest numbers of refugees from that region came from Vietnam, and there were also significant numbers from Cambodia and Laos. In the 1990s the greatest numbers of refugees, besides those from Southeast Asia, were from the former Soviet Union, and beginning in the 2000s the largest percentage of refugees to the United States has come from the Near East and South Asia (Refugee Processing Center 2016). Refugees from these countries included those from Afghanistan, Iraq, Iran, and Myanmar, and refugees from Bhutan who had been resettled in other parts of South Asia.

In the 2000s refugees to the United States also have come from Latin America and the Caribbean. These countries include primarily Guatemala, El Salvador, Honduras, Cuba, and Haiti. In the 2000s refugees also began coming from various parts of Central and East Africa, including the Democratic Republic of the Congo, Sudan, Ethiopia, Eritrea, and Somalia (Refugee Processing Center 2016).

Because of changes in the U.S. government's policy toward admission of refugees, there has been a decline over the last few years in the number of refugees authorized to enter the United States. For example, in fiscal year 2016, there were approximately 85,000 refugees admitted to the United States, but in fiscal year 2017 there were only about 54,000, with the approval ceiling for 2018 being less than that number (Refugee Health Technical Assistance Center 2011). Of the refugees admitted to the United States in fiscal year 2017, the largest number were from Africa (approximately 20,000) and from the Near East and South Asia (also approximately 20,000). Refugees from Somalia and the Democratic Republic of the Congo accounted for the majority of arrivals from Africa. From the Near East and South Asia, the majority of refugees were from Iraq, Syria, and Bhutan (Refugee Processing Center 2016).

The conditions in the countries that have produced the largest number of refugees who have come to the United States in the last several years mirror the conditions that have produced refugees during the latter part of the twentieth century and the first decade of this century. There continues to be great instability in the Near East due to continued war, and these conditions show no signs of disappearing. In addition, there have been numerous civil wars in Central and East Africa, complicated by significant climate stressors such as severe drought, that have contributed to disease and malnutrition. As in so many areas of the world from which refugees come, a combination of conditions, such as war, environmental degradation, and collapse of civil society, creates very unstable conditions that lead to further violence and further shortages of food, water, and basic health care that have an impact on the population.

The significant majority of people migrating from the Central American countries of El Salvador, Guatemala, and Honduras have not been screened for official refugee status; they have come as undocumented migrants, many of whom have applied for asylum. Those applying for asylum have not been legally approved for residency in the United States. There are two routes to gaining asylum, affirmatively through the U.S. Citizenship and Immigration Services, or defensively through an immigration judge as part of a removal proceeding. The affirmative channel is open to applicants regardless of whether they have entered the country legally (De Jesús-Rentas et al. 2010). Many asylum seekers from Central America in recent years have also been unaccompanied minors fleeing violence and instability in their countries. El Salvador and Guatemala both experienced civil wars during the 1980s and 1990s, and postwar instability has continued because of gang violence, much of which is tied to the drug trade throughout the Americas. Children, particularly males, have been pressured to join gangs and to participate in horrendous violence that is part of the background of daily life in these countries. Many violent events are not reported to the police because of fear of police corruption or gang-related retaliation (Keller et al. 2017). To escape inscription into gangs, minors often leave on their own or with the encouragement of their families to seek safety in the United States. Both youth and adult migrants from these Central American countries must come through Mexico and then cross the United States–Mexican border under very difficult climatic and environmental conditions, and after being subjected to various forms of exploitation while traveling through Mexico.

ARRIVAL IN THE UNITED STATES

The cities and states where refugees are resettled frequently do not have similarities of climate or size to the areas from which they came. Resettlement is often dependent on sponsorship by nongovernmental organizations, religious communities, and other local and state agencies. After arriving in the United States, refugees and asylum seekers often migrate to various parts of the country after their initial resettlement. This secondary migration within the United States is sometimes driven by refugees wanting to join extended family in different parts of the country or to pursue job opportunities that may not be available where they originally settled.

Now that I have outlined the demographic characteristics of refugees who have resettled in the United States and described the conditions across the globe that produce refugees, I would like to summarize the epidemiological findings over the last several decades relating to mental health conditions among refugees. After summarizing these data, I then discuss current recommended approaches to assessment and treatment, which will be described in more detail in the chapters that follow.

PSYCHIATRIC CONDITIONS AMONG REFUGEES

Because of the conditions that refugees experience during the various stages of migration, there are certain psychiatric conditions that are more prevalent than others. However, among refugee populations there are certain conditions that are encountered in any population seeking psychiatric treatment. These include a range of psychotic, mood, and anxiety disorders. As with any population, refugees are at risk for cognitive disorders such as dementia, but because of exposure to violence and traumatic brain injury, they may be more at risk for cognitive disorders as they age. A combination of biological, psychological, and social factors, in addition to the complex interplay of migration, cultural bereavement, and threats to cultural identity, plays a significant role in rates of mental illness in migrant groups (Bhugra and Becker 2005). Proper use of diagnostic methods is a key step in assessing cross-cultural factors related to epidemiology, etiology of illness, prognosis, and treatment in the context of the sociocultural milieu in which the refugee patient functions and is essential for distinguishing psychopathology from abnormal behavior (Westermeyer 1987). It is also essential that the diagnostic process allow for variations in cultural background, including sensitivity to cultural values, religious beliefs, and social structure, in conceptualizing and treating symptoms and restoring the patient to health (Boehnlein and Kinzie 1997).

Despite the conditions that refugees experience prior to resettlement, there currently is no clear evidence that the prevalence rates of mental disorders among refugees in the initial years of resettlement are significantly higher or lower than those in the host population (Giacco and Priebe 2018), with the exception of psychosis and PTSD (Kirkbride 2017). However, over the long term, among resettled refugees, the rates of depression and anxiety disorders seem to be higher than those in the host populations, while the rates of PTSD continue to be higher than those in the host populations (Bogic et al. 2015).

Torture is a particularly prominent risk factor for the development of PTSD among refugees (Steel et al. 2009), and accumulative exposure to multiple types of torture predicts anxiety and PTSD (Song et al. 2018). It is important to note that refugees cannot be regarded as a homogeneous group, so generalized statements concerning prevalence rates of mental disorders among refugees also need to be interpreted with some caution (Giacco and Priebe 2018; Hollander et al. 2016). As an example of cross-cultural variability in certain types of psychiatric conditions, even though PTSD has substantial cross-cultural validity, there can be substantial variability in the prevalence of specific symptom clusters, particularly avoidance and somatic symptoms (Hinton and Lewis-Fernández 2011).

The level of threat that a community may continue to face after resettlement, and other postmigration stressors, all make major contributions to the prevalence of disorders among refugee populations (Silove et al. 2017). Other postdisplacement factors, such as living in institutional accommodations or having restricted economic opportunities, are associated with worse outcomes (Porter and Haslam 2005). In addition, the length of time after resettlement before mental health services are accessed is an important factor associated with depression and PTSD symptoms, after adjustment for other pre- and postmigration social factors, including torture and psychosocial stress (Song et al. 2015). Another environmental condition affecting the prevalence of disorders among refugees is residing in refugee camps in low-income countries, which is associated with a high prevalence of anxiety and depression that reflects the highly stressful conditions typically encountered in refugee camps (Hynie 2018). This risk factor is related to time elapsed before mental health services are accessed (Song et al. 2018).

Besides the ongoing risks of trauma postresettlement, other factors that have been identified as being associated with poor mental health outcomes among refugees include unemployment, discrimination, and limited acquisition of language skills that are necessary for optimal functioning in the host country (Kim 2016). Conversely, stable and uncrowded housing has been found to predict lower rates of PTSD, depression, and anxiety symptoms after resettlement (Whitsett and Sherman 2017). Ongoing separation from family members in the country of origin has been found to be a significant risk factor for poor refugee mental health postresettlement (Miller et al. 2018). Family separation contributes to ill health because of ongoing fears for the safety of family members still in harm's way in the country of origin and a feeling of powerlessness to assist those family members. Finally, demographic factors that have been shown to be consistently associated with mental ill health among refugees are gender (women at higher risk), age (elderly at higher risk), and divorced or being widowed (Tinghög et al. 2017).

Comorbidity of conditions is important in any discussion of psychiatric conditions among refugees. PTSD and depression are highly comorbid in refugee populations, and the symptoms of each cumulatively add to distress. In addition, refugees who have been exposed to violence and physical injury, particularly those who have experienced interpersonal trauma such as torture, are also at increased risk for traumatic brain injury. Comorbid traumatic brain injury and PTSD can be additive in impairing postoptimal functioning, and they commonly have overlapping symptoms. Related to risk factors for refugee mental health, as the number of trauma and torture events increases concurrently with increases in traumatic brain injury, the presence of depression and PTSD also increases (Mollica et al. 2014). Refugees with comorbid PTSD and severe depression have been found to not benefit as much from treatment for PTSD when the depression is not adequately addressed (Haagen et al. 2017). Another comorbid condition affecting outcome of depression and PTSD among refugees is chronic pain, which can be the result of injuries suffered premigration and during the migration process. This is particularly important for those who have experienced interpersonal violence and torture. Assessment of other physical health conditions is also important. For example, refugees with comorbid PTSD and depression have been found to have an increased prevalence of physical health problems, such as hypertension and diabetes, compared with those without either of those conditions (Berthold et al. 2014).

ASSESSMENT OF REFUGEE MENTAL HEALTH IN THE CLINICAL SETTING

It is important that refugees referred for psychiatric assessment and treatment receive a comprehensive assessment rather than one focusing exclusively on recent events and stressors. A comprehensive assessment includes a complete developmental history of the refugee's childhood experiences and an assessment of developmental milestones and any evidence of childhood illnesses that may affect cognitive and psychological functioning. The examiner rarely has any records from the patient's country of origin, and frequently there is no collateral information available, but it is still important to gain as much information as possible. It is important to ask about a history of head injury, loss of consciousness, or other types of physical trauma that the person may have experienced as a child or adolescent. In addition, an assessment of the patient's home environment, including key attachment figures, is very important, particularly because refugees have so frequently suffered numerous disruptions to important attachment figures throughout their lives, including recent separation from loved ones.

From a psychiatric perspective, it is important to connect any significant losses or disruptions of attachment experienced in childhood to psychological and emotional challenges that the patient may be facing in his or her life postmigration. Such connections are also particularly relevant to the relationship between the patient and the clinician. Many refugees have had difficult experiences with authority figures in their native countries, and, in addition, the health screening procedures prior to their resettlement may have been rushed and impersonal. Therefore, it will take time for the individual to develop some trust in the mental health assessment and treatment process because previously painful experiences of loss or disruption of trust in key attachment figures during early development or early adulthood may affect the person's ability to develop trust. Moreover, expressing one's painful history and emotions fully may be additionally challenging when there is an interpreter involved in the assessment process.

Besides the presence of an interpreter during the assessment, it is important for the examiner to also be aware of variations in nonverbal behavior that occur cross culturally. The examiner may falsely interpret a flat affect as being a sign of depression or disinterest, when it may actually be a sign of trepidation or hesitation on the part of the patient. Because of shame or stigma, refugee patients also may underplay the severity of their symptoms or the pain associated with their distress, and may project themselves as being healthier than they actually are. There also may be expectations within the person's culture that discourage the sharing of intense emotions or very personal feelings associated with sadness, depression, or loss. In addition, the person may be hesitant to share frightening experiences and perceptions that may be psychotic in nature, such as hallucinations, because of fear of being labeled as mentally ill. Being aware of cultural idioms of distress is important for the clinician's ability to respond to patient and family concerns and to reduce the risk of stigmatization (Bäärnhielm et al. 2017; Kinzie et al. 1997). Moreover, ascribing mental health symptoms to culturally acceptable terms can provide individuals with a less stigmatized way of discussing their mental health needs (Im et al. 2017).

The psychiatric assessment of a refugee patient should include all the other important standard elements of a psychiatric assessment, including the history, severity, and time course of the current symptoms. It should also include a past medical and psychiatric history and a family history of medical and psychiatric conditions. The latter is often difficult to assess because of the patient's frequent lack of knowledge of medical and psychiatric conditions that were experienced in previous generations, particularly if certain conditions have a great deal of stigma attached to them. Because of the comorbidity of several conditions that are frequently found in refugee populations such as PTSD, depression, and traumatic brain injury, it is important to obtain a more detailed history of patterns of insomnia, headache, pain, and other frequently reported physical complaints. Stress may frequently be communicated through physical complaints such as headache, joint, and limb pain. Differential diagnosis of headache, which is a common chief complaint among refugees with PTSD and depression, is quite broad and includes tension, migraine, and posttraumatic headaches. Insomnia is a presenting symptom that can allow for an expanded discussion of important experiences that the refugee patient may have difficulty spontaneously discussing, such as previous traumatic experiences that are replayed in nightmares. Severe insomnia, often associated with recurrent nightmares, adds to the disability that is associated with depression and can contribute to significant difficulties with daytime functioning and the fulfillment of family and social responsibilities. The proper assessment of insomnia and associated nightmares can allow for early specific medication and psychotherapy treatment interventions that can significantly alleviate disabling symptoms in a short period of time, and contribute to increased functioning, enhanced trust in the provider, and optimal adherence with treatment.

The psychosocial segment of the psychiatric assessment should include a history of the patient's premigration experiences, migratory experiences, and the stressors currently encountered in the host country. This section of the assessment can draw on important elements from the Cultural Formulation Interview Supplementary Module for Refugees (Boehnlein et al. 2015). The interviewer does not have to literally follow each question in the cultural formulation interview; rather, he or she can integrate various elements into a narrative assessment. Some questions that can be helpful include asking patients when and with whom did they leave their home country, how many family members remain, and whether they have particular concerns about family members who remain there. In addition, the examiner can ask the patient about his or her reasons for leaving the home country and ask about losses that he or she experienced before leaving, including the possible deaths of family members or close friends, and the loss of homes and property, livelihood, and education opportunities. At this point further into the interview, when the patient may be more relaxed and trusting, the examiner can ask the patient about possible experiences of violence or other trauma that he or she had experienced in the home country or during the process of migration. The examiner can also ask about the most formidable challenges the patient has faced since arriving in the host country and what types of fears and hopes the patient may have about his or her current and future life, including stability of income, housing, and employment, and prospects for education. Additionally, it is important to ask about the current family constellation and about challenges experienced within the family cross-generationally and with possible new roles for various members of the family.

Additional questions are important in a comprehensive assessment. How might cultural issues be impeding or enhancing the individual and the family's acculturation and settlement in their new country? What are their sources of support such as other extended family, church, or friends? What are sources of meaning and hope? What strengths and talents does the person have? Finally, what is the individual's expectations for treatment, and what difficulties or symptoms are he or she most interested in reducing during treatment? The clinician can then proceed to a differential diagnosis and formulation of the patient's difficulties that includes a comprehensive view of biological, psychological, and social and cultural factors that have an impact on the patient's symptom presentation, emotional suffering, and current functioning.

GENERAL ISSUES IN THE TREATMENT OF REFUGEE PATIENTS

Because of the heterogeneity of refugee populations, effective treatment requires attention to broad demographic differences and a wide range of disorders for which refugees seek care. There are barriers to access, such as language, long travel distances for care, lack of knowledge about treatment options, and lack of familiarity with the American health care system (Sijbrandij 2018). Other barriers to access include economic factors, health literacy, and various cultural factors that affect the understanding of treatment options and the perception of mental illness within refugee communities (Mangrio and Sjögren Forss 2017).

Differences in expectations between refugee communities and the American health care system involving the causes and meaning of symptoms and illness can be just as important as other barriers to care. Understanding how the mind and body function; what role various cultural healing traditions, religious systems, and social structures may be playing; how one communicates distress; and how the patient views the causes of his or her distress are key factors in designing affective treatment and optimizing adherence (Hinton and Lewis-Fernández 2011). Errors in diagnosis, of course, can have a significant impact on the choice of effective treatments. For example, in treating psychosis cross-culturally, errors can occur in clinical misunderstanding of symptoms that appear to be psychotic, such as interpreting a cultural belief as a delusion or a trance state as a hallucination. Also, the presence of multiple diagnoses, such as the coexistence of PTSD and depression commonly found in refugee populations, may require a variety of long-term interventions to address the pervasive effects of illness on the refugee's distress, social functioning, and quality of life (Nickerson et al. 2017). The effectiveness of mental health interventions during refugee resettlement depends on not only how well those interventions alleviate symptoms of psychosis, depression, or PTSD, but also how well those interventions relate directly to educational, socioeconomic, and sociopolitical stressors that resettled refugees encounter (Murray et al. 2010). The importance of these contextual factors—and in particular exposure to significant postmigration stress—can further reinforce PTSD and depression among refugees.

Strengthening of social networks and supports, and the strengthening of other postmigration contextual factors such as employment, can provide protective effects (Beiser and Hou 2017; Paat and Green 2017). Because of the complex trauma experienced by many refugees, it is important for the treatment setting to create a trusting environment that is sensitive to difficulties that patients may have with attachment and trust (Morina et al. 2016; Riber 2017). Overall, treatment of refugees in mental health settings could be enhanced by the ADAPT model, which postulates that stable societies are built on five core psychosocial pillars disrupted by mass conflict: safety/security, bonds/networks, identity/roles, justice, and existential meaning (Silove 2013).

Most treatment studies among refugee populations have demonstrated significant improvement on at least one outcome indicator after treatment interventions. But there have been very few randomized controlled trials that have examined the efficacy of applied treatments, and they have included only small samples. This paucity of large outcome studies and randomized controlled trials among refugees is likely due to a number of factors, such as the heterogeneity of refugee populations, the difficulties of using validated treatments across cultures, the mobility of the refugee populations, and ethical issues in effectively studying traumatized populations, and applies to studies that examine psychopharmacological as well as psychotherapeutic interventions for refugees. Because there is very limited evidence available from controlled trials on the effectiveness of psychopharmacological agents in refugee populations with PTSD, clinicians depend on a combination of clinical experience and research results from trials in nonrefugee populations (Sonne et al. 2017). From the standpoint of psychotherapy, taken together, studies support the use of some form of trauma-focused cognitive-behavioral therapy (CBT) among refugees that incorporate cultural knowledge into standard CBT methods (Slobodin and de Jong 2015).

There continues to be controversy over what constitutes effective culturally adapted psychotherapy for refugee populations. For example, narrative exposure therapy, a manualized variant of CBT with a trauma focus, has been shown in meta-analyses to be the best supported intervention (Nosè et al. 2017), but the evidence is based on studies of mostly low methodological quality and small to medium effect sizes (Giacco and

Priebe 2018). Culturally adapted CBT has been found to be a significantly effective treatment for PTSD and panic attacks among Vietnamese refugees (Hinton et al. 2004) and for PTSD and associated symptoms in Cambodian refugees (Otto et al. 2003). In the latter study the effectiveness of CBT was felt to be particularly effective in addressing catastrophic misinterpretations of culturally relevant symptoms.

The psychotherapeutic relationship can offer cognitive and emotional generosity to refugee patients to titrate their anxiety and to help them find coherence and trust (Kirmayer 2003). From the very beginning of treatment, it is important for clinicians to focus on relieving symptoms that will improve practical individual and interpersonal functioning. As stated earlier, these symptoms may extend to a number of diagnostic categories, such as depression, PTSD, other anxiety disorders, and psychosis. Many of the symptoms that patients initially describe that cause significant suffering and interpersonal dysfunction can also provide a window into other intense struggles that these patients may be having. As mentioned, insomnia may not only be distressing but have significant effects on daytime functioning, along with a sense of security and confidence in work and interpersonal relationships. Nightmares can provide a window into psychological struggles that the patient may be having, and this marker can be a potential marker for success of treatment. The intensity and frequency of nightmares can be reduced by prazosin or clonidine (Boehnlein and Kinzie 2007). The discussion between the survivor and the clinician of nightmare content and the accompanying emotional reactions humanizes the therapeutic encounter. And, the discussion of pain, loss, heartache, and struggle allows for a longitudinal consideration of issues vital to recovery that otherwise might be avoided by the clinician and survivor.

Education of the patient and family is vitally important, particularly in terms of being able to discuss common posttraumatic symptoms in order to reduce personal and social stigma. Reducing hyperarousal symptoms such as nightmares with effective medication can allow the person to more readily engage interpersonally and socially and also benefit more fully from psychotherapy and social intervention. Helping the survivor to process and integrate current and past trauma and interpersonal challenges can increase self-confidence and allow the person to more fully concentrate on a brighter and more promising future, further increasing the sense of well-being.

Besides various symptoms that refugees experience individually, families collectively confront numerous stressful challenges in resettlement that may alter the traditional structure of the family and may provide further challenges for acculturation. For example, after migration, older refugees may have to live with diminished status both within families and in society at large because of a lack of language proficiency, little or no formal education, and no work skills for urban developed countries. As children gain greater proficiency with the host country language, there can be a reversal of traditional generational roles as the children become facilitators of communication and culture brokers between the family and the majority of society. Even normal life-cycle separations for family members can present additional challenges for refugee families. For example, because of the extensive loss of life that many families have experienced, they may be more adversely affected by culturally expected separations in Western society, such as a child's leaving the house for college or moving to another part of the country after marriage for greater employment opportunities.

Chronic depression and PTSD can adversely affect the stability and nurturance of family relationships. Family therapy with refugee families can help restore cultural identity that was lost or weakened during the years of trauma and migration, and also reduce the pressures of acculturation. This latter task may include helping each generation to understand and accept one another's beliefs and roles as the family evolves through the life cycle in the new society. In addition, treatment can incorporate the strengths that allowed all members to survive individually and as a unit (Boehnlein et al. 1997). Adequately addressing trust in self, others, and the world that has been disrupted by trauma and forced migration is an essential core of treatment for refugees of all generations (Ter Heide et al. 2017). Such trust building is ideally done not just through traditional culturally sensitive mental health services, but through an array of services that include social and community interventions and special programs for vulnerable refugee groups (Silove et al. 2017). A phased approach can be especially helpful, beginning with first establishing emotional and social safety and security, followed by psychosocial interventions such as enhancing skills that optimize education and employment opportunities (Rousseau 2017). For refugee children, this would include optimizing family and parenting support, along with school-based interventions (Fazel 2018).

CASE EXAMPLE

In this chapter I have explored general aspects of refugee mental health assessment and treatment; details of various treatment approaches are discussed in more detail in the chapters that follow. The following case provides a clinical context for several issues discussed in this introductory chapter, and subsequent chapters, that are central to refugee mental health.

A 42-year-old widowed Guatemalan woman was referred to the clinic by her immigration attorney. Several months before her initial clinic evaluation, an extended family member was killed in Guatemala and her family there was threatened by people connected to the government during the civil war. The patient stated in the initial evaluation that she thinks about the past every day and is worried about the future. She was chronically anxious, and for years she had not been able to trust other people. Since arrival in the United States she also had felt anxious and angry when she saw military or police uniforms, thinking to herself that they were murderers just like the Guatemalan military who had killed her husband. She was sleeping only 2–3 hours at night and had chronic and recurrent nightmares that were also regularly associated with daytime intrusive trauma memories. Her nightmares centered around her husband's murder, the exact reenactment of another murder that she witnessed in her neighborhood in Guatemala, and her sexual assault while crossing the Mexico–United States border. She also reported startle reactions and frequent headaches associated with intrusive memories and worry, and she experienced isolation, sadness, and irritability. She avoided all violence in the media and any interpersonal situations in which people were raising their voices or confronting each other.

The patient grew up in northern Guatemala in the Mayan area of the country. Her parents were farmers, and she had three brothers and two sisters. There was no violence or abuse within the family. When she was growing up, her family was frequently moving because of hostilities in their area of the country. They were constantly caught between the military and guerrillas and were frequently accused by the military of aiding the guerrillas. Food products were often withheld from the family or intercepted by the military, so there was a great deal of deprivation.

During the initial few months of treatment with an antidepressant and prazosin, her sleep improved and the frequency of her nightmares decreased to a couple of nights per week. After 4 months, her sleep returned to normal and her mood gradually improved. Six months after treatment began she was granted asylum and her nightmares decreased to a frequency of twice per month. However, during the damp winter months her nightmares temporarily increased in frequency every year, and she herself noted that it was likely related to seasonal reminders of the dampness in her native area of Guatemala, and to traumatic war memories, including the winter murder of her husband. The etiology and seasonal context of these nightmares were discussed in follow-up treatment sessions. During several years of treatment she functioned very well during most of the year, and her yearly anniversary reaction gradually decreased in intensity and duration during the course of treatment.

KEY CLINICAL POINTS

The following are some important issues for clinicians to keep in mind when they are working with refugee patients and families:

- Validate and normalize difficulties in transition and resettlement.
- Be aware of the impact of loss and the fragility of relationships both in the host country and country of origin, particularly in patients with depression and PTSD.
- Be aware of dynamics and interactive patterns of family, cultural, and religious values/beliefs.
- Assess the degree of family cohesion, social and gender role transitions, extended family and social support networks, and strengths.
- Determine the degree of acculturation of each family member—don't assume the degree of acculturation on the basis of age, gender, or level of education.
- Be aware of one's own biases, blind spots, and strengths as a person and clinician.

REFERENCES

Administration for Children and Families: Refugee Act of 1980. Office of Refugee Resettlement. 2012. Available at: https://www.acf.hhs.gov/orr/resource/the-refugee-act. Accessed October 7, 2019.

Administration for Children and Families: Training and technical assistance providers. 2019. Office of Refugee Resettlement. Available at: https://www.acf.hhs.gov/orr/resource/technical-assistance-providers-1. Accessed October 7, 2019.

Bäärnhielm S, Laban K, Schouler-Ocak M, et al: Mental health for refugees, asylum seekers and displaced persons: a call for a humanitarian agenda. Transcult Psychiatry 54(5–6):565–574, 2017 29226788

Beiser M, Hou F: Predictors of positive mental health among refugees: Results from Canada's General Social Survey. Transcult Psychiatry 54(5–6):675–695, 2017 28854860

Berthold SM, Kong S, Mollica RF, et al: Comorbid mental and physical health and health access in Cambodian refugees in the US. J Community Health 39(6):1045–1052, 2014 24651944

Bhugra D, Becker MA: Migration, cultural bereavement and cultural identity. World Psychiatry 4(1):18–24, 2005 16633496

Boehnlein JK, Kinzie JD: Cultural perspectives on posttraumatic stress disorder, in Clinical Disorders and Stressful Life Events. Edited by Miller TW. Madison, CT, International Universities Press, 1997, pp 19–43

Boehnlein JK, Kinzie JD: Pharmacologic reduction of CNS noradrenergic activity in PTSD: the case for clonidine and prazosin. J Psychiatr Pract 13(2):72–78, 2007 17414682

Boehnlein JK, Leung PK, Kinzie JD: Cambodian American families, in Working With Asian Americans: A Guide for Clinicians. Edited by Lee E. New York, Guilford, 1997, pp 37–45

Boehnlein JK, Westermeyer J, Scalco M: The cultural formulation interview for refugees and immigrants, in DSM-5 Handbook on the Cultural Formulation Interview. Edited by Lewis-Fernandez R, Aggarwal N, Hinton L, et al. Washington DC, American Psychiatric Publishing, 2015, pp 173–181

Bogic M, Njoku A, Priebe S: Long-term mental health of war-refugees: a systematic literature review. BMC Int Health Hum Rights 15:29, 2015 26510473

De Jesús-Rentas G, Boehnlein J, Sparr L: Central American victims of gang violence as asylum seekers: the role of the forensic expert. J Am Acad Psychiatry Law 38(4):490–498, 2010 21156907

Fazel M: Psychological and psychosocial interventions for refugee children resettled in high-income countries. Epidemiol Psychiatr Sci 27(2):117–123, 2018 29122044

Giacco D, Priebe S: Mental health care for adult refugees in high-income countries. Epidemiol Psychiatr Sci 27(2):109–116, 2018 29067899

Haagen JFG, Ter Heide FJJ, Mooren TM, et al: Predicting post-traumatic stress disorder treatment response in refugees: multilevel analysis. Br J Clin Psychol 56(1):69–83, 2017 27900778

Hinton DE, Lewis-Fernández R: The cross-cultural validity of posttraumatic stress disorder: implications for DSM-5. Depress Anxiety 28(9):783–801, 2011 21910185

Hinton DE, Pham T, Tran M, et al: CBT for Vietnamese refugees with treatment-resistant PTSD and panic attacks: a pilot study. J Trauma Stress 17(5):429–433, 2004 15633922

Hollander AC, Dal H, Lewis G, et al: Refugee migration and risk of schizophrenia and other non-affective psychoses: cohort study of 1.3 million people in Sweden. BMJ 352:i1030, 2016 26979256

Hynie M: The social determinants of refugee mental health in the post-migration context: a critical review. Can J Psychiatry 63(5):297–303, 2018 29202665

Im H, Ferguson A, Hunter M: Cultural translation of refugee trauma: cultural idioms of distress among Somali refugees in displacement. Transcult Psychiatry 54(5–6):626–652, 2017 29226793

Keller A, Joscelyne A, Granski M, et al: Pre-migration trauma exposure and mental health functioning among Central American migrants arriving at the US border. PLoS One 12(1):e0168692, 2017 28072836

Kim I: Beyond trauma: post-resettlement factors and mental health outcomes among Latino and Asian refugees in the United States. J Immigr Minor Health 18(4):740–748, 2016 26169507

Kinzie JD, Leung PK, Boehnlein JK: Treatment of depressive disorders in refugees, in Working With Asian Americans: A Guide for Clinicians. Edited by Lee E. New York, Guilford, 1997, pp 265–274

Kirkbride JB: Migration and psychosis: our smoking lung? World Psychiatry 16(2):119–120, 2017 28498570

Kirmayer LJ: Failures of imagination: the refugee's narrative in psychiatry. Anthropol Med 10(2):167–185, 2003 26954835

Mangrio E, Sjögren Forss K: Refugees' experiences of healthcare in the host country: a scoping review. BMC Health Serv Res 17(1):814, 2017 29216876

Miller A, Hess JM, Bybee D, et al: Understanding the mental health consequences of family separation for refugees: implications for policy and practice. Am J Orthopsychiatry 88(1):26–37, 2018 28617002

Mollica RF, Chernoff MC, Megan Berthold S, et al: The mental health sequelae of traumatic head injury in South Vietnamese ex-political detainees who survived torture. Compr Psychiatry 55(7):1626–1638, 2014 24962448

Morina N, Schnyder U, Schick M, et al: Attachment style and interpersonal trauma in refugees. Aust N Z J Psychiatry 50(12):1161–1168, 2016 26883572

Murray KE, Davidson GR, Schweitzer RD: Review of refugee mental health interventions following resettlement: best practices and recommendations. Am J Orthopsychiatry 80(4):576–585, 2010 20950298

Nickerson A, Schick M, Schnyder U, et al: Comorbidity of posttraumatic stress disorder and depression in tortured, treatment-seeking refugees. J Trauma Stress 30(4):409–415, 2017 28763568

Nosè M, Ballette F, Bighelli I, et al: Psychosocial interventions for post-traumatic stress disorder in refugees and asylum seekers resettled in high-income countries: Systematic review and meta-analysis. PLoS One 12(2):e0171030, 2017 28151992

Otto MW, Hinton D, Korbly NB, et al: Treatment of pharmacotherapy-refractory posttraumatic stress disorder among Cambodian refugees: a pilot study of combination treatment with cognitive-behavior therapy vs sertraline alone. Behav Res Ther 41(11):1271–1276, 2003 14527527

Paat YF, Green R: Mental health of immigrants and refugees seeking legal services on the US-Mexico border. Transcult Psychiatry 54(5–6):783–805, 2017 29226794

Porter M, Haslam N: Predisplacement and postdisplacement factors associated with mental health of refugees and internally displaced persons: a meta-analysis. JAMA 294(5):602–612, 2005 16077055

Refugee Health Technical Assistance Center: Refugee resettlement. 2011. Available at: http://refugeehealthta.org/refugee-basics/refugee-resettlement. Accessed October 7, 2019.

Refugee Processing Center: Admission and arrivals. 2016. Available at: https://www.wrapsnet.org/admissions-and-arrivals. Accessed October 7, 2019.

Riber K: Trauma complexity and child abuse: A qualitative study of attachment narratives in adult refugees with PTSD. Transcult Psychiatry 54(5–6):840–869, 2017 29130379

Rousseau C: Addressing mental health needs of refugees. Can J Psychiatry 63(5):287–289, 2017 29202662

Sijbrandij M: Expanding the evidence: key priorities for research on mental health interventions for refugees in high-income countries. Epidemiol Psychiatr Sci 27(2):105–108, 2018 29143713

Silove D: The ADAPT model: a conceptual framework for mental health and psychosocial programming in post conflict settings. Intervention (Amstelveen) 11:237–248, 2013

Silove D, Ventevogel P, Rees S: The contemporary refugee crisis: an overview of mental health challenges. World Psychiatry 16(2):130–139, 2017 28498581

Slobodin O, de Jong JT: Mental health interventions for traumatized asylum seekers and refugees: What do we know about their efficacy? Int J Soc Psychiatry 61(1):17–26, 2015 24869847

Song SJ, Kaplan C, Tol WA, et al: Psychological distress in torture survivors: pre- and post-migration risk factors in a US sample. Soc Psychiatry Psychiatr Epidemiol 50(4):549–560, 2015 25403567

Song SJ, Subica A, Kaplan C, et al: Predicting the mental health and functioning of torture survivors. J Nerv Ment Dis 206(1):33–39, 2018 28350563

Sonne C, Carlsson J, Bech P, et al: Pharmacological treatment of refugees with trauma-related disorders: What do we know today? Transcult Psychiatry 54(2):260–280, 2017 27956478

Steel Z, Chey T, Silove D, et al: Association of torture and other potentially traumatic events with mental health outcomes among populations exposed to mass conflict and displacement: a systematic review and meta-analysis. JAMA 302(5):537–549, 2009 19654388

Ter Heide FJJ, Sleijpen M, van der Aa N: Posttraumatic world assumptions among treatment-seeking refugees. Transcult Psychiatry 54(5–6):824–839, 2017 29226792

Tinghög P, Malm A, Arwidson C, et al: Prevalence of mental ill health, traumas and postmigration stress among refugees from Syria resettled in Sweden after 2011: a population-based survey. BMJ Open 7(12):e018899, 2017 29289940

United Nations High Commission for Refugees: The 1951 Convention and Its 1967 Protocol Relating to the Status of Refugees. September 2011. Available at: http://www.unhcr.org/en-us/about-us/background/4ec262df9/1951-convention-relating-status-refugees-its-1967-protocol.html. Accessed October 7, 2019.

United Nations High Commissioner for Refugees: Figures at a glance. 2019.
    Available at: http://www.unhcr.org/figures-at-a-glance.html. Accessed
    October 7, 2019.
Westermeyer J: Clinical considerations in cross-cultural diagnosis. Hosp Com-
    munity Psychiatry 38(2):160–165, 1987 3557340
Whitsett D, Sherman MF: Do resettlement variables predict psychiatric treat-
    ment outcomes in a sample of asylum-seeking survivors of torture? Int J
    Soc Psychiatry 63(8):674–685, 2017 28838279

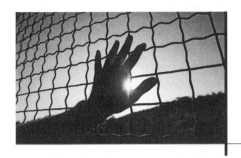

Chapter 2

DIAGNOSIS AND TREATMENT

J. David Kinzie, M.D., FACPsych, DLFAPA

DIAGNOSTIC PROCESS OF REFUGEE PATIENTS

The following is a diagnostic interview, conducted by the author, with a refugee patient. Prior to the interview I had a little knowledge of the patient. I knew that she was Cambodian and that her age meant that she had experienced the genocide of the Pol Pot regime. The interview was done with my counselor Ben, a Cambodian who had worked with me for 15 years at the time of the interview. The information is mixed with my own comments and recollections of the interaction. The interview is characterized by two people, a psychiatrist and his patient, who do not know each other and who are establishing a relationship. The interview proceeded in a slow deliberate fashion and took about 90 minutes.

Background of the Pol Pot Regime in Cambodia

In 1975, Pol Pot led a group of teen-age guerillas to take over Cambodia. His goal was to establish an extreme form of peasant communism. The movement was an attempt to destroy all forms of previous "corrupt" influences of the "old ways." This meant that people associated with city life, religion, and Western ideas—Buddhist monks, doctors, lawyers, military members—were subject to execution. Families were placed in work communities, where they were forced to work from 4 A.M.

to 10 P.M. with little rest and very little food. Children were often separated from parents and placed in groups with other children. Twenty-five percent of the population of eight million died of starvation, disease, or execution. The regime ended in 1978 when the Vietnamese invaded the country (The History Place 1999).

This much was known to me through available reports at the time on the subject. However, by the time of the interview of "Sok" (not her real name to protect confidentiality), I had heard probably 50 reports with very similar stories. Working with this patient emphasizes the importance of knowing something about the situation in the country from where the refugee came. Most refugees left their countries because of genocide, ethnic cleansing, persecution, death of family members, or threats of being killed themselves. It is necessary to understand this in order to begin the interview with some empathy for what they have been through.

The Interview

I introduced myself to the patient and asked her her name. She said, "Sok." I then asked her what her main problems were. She gave a history of having trouble concentrating, very poor sleep, depression, low energy, poor memory, and, at times, suicidal thoughts and behavior. She had overdosed in the past, about 6 months before the time of the interview. Every night she would have nightmares, which were about the events that occurred in Cambodia. She had increased anger and avoidance of all violence, especially that depicted on television. The symptoms had increased since her boyfriend left her after she became pregnant. She described no psychotic symptoms. She had no medical problems, and her blood pressure was normal.

After obtaining the history of Sok's symptoms of the present illness, I began taking a chronological history of her life starting when she was young. She was born and raised in a rural area of Cambodia. Her parents had eight children; three died young and five remained alive. Her father was in the military, and the mother worked on their farm. The patient also worked on the farm for several years, and she only attended school 2–3 years.

At this point, I asked what had happened to her during the Pol Pot time. She described much fear and starvation. Her father was killed in front of her. She was forced to marry but never saw her new husband after a short time. Both of her brothers were in battles and killed, but she could not give any details. In the community commune, she was caught stealing food, tied up, and beaten. She was told that she would be killed in the morning, but she was saved. She had a child and escaped to Thailand when the Vietnamese invaded. She stayed in Thailand for 2 years. Her description of the events of the Pol Pot regime was given briefly and without detail. However, she displayed sadness and crying as she described the death of her father, and also being alone with her baby.

In the United States she had a boyfriend for 2 years who was abusive and beat her. While she was pregnant with her second child, she took an overdose and was hospitalized. She was unsure if life was worth living now.

At this point in the interview, it was clear there was enough evidence to make a diagnosis of PTSD and major depressive disorder. What was needed was for me to give some information to the patient and for us to provide hope for the future. I said, "You are a very strong person, but even a strong person breaks down. Many terrible things happened to you—watching your father being killed, two brothers being killed; being starved; and being threatened with death and abused by men. Now having a child and another one on the way." I asked her if there was anything else in the story that I had missed or if there was any other thing she wanted to say. She said no.

After inquiring about all the symptoms she mentioned—poor concentration, insomnia, nightmares, anger, avoidance behavior—I asked, "What is the most troublesome that we should work on?" She said she would like to sleep better and would like to have help with the nightmares. I told her that I could help with the sleep, nightmares, and the depression but that I could not take away the many losses and the sense of abandonment she has endured. Medicine would not take them away but could diminish some of their impact.

I asked her to commit to three things in our treatment: 1) She must take the medicine as prescribed, 2) she must keep her appointments, and 3) she must not kill herself. Looking her directly, I asked, "Do you agree to this?" and she said, "Yes." I explained that the medicine would help—that it had some side effects, but she would be able to sleep better, the nightmares would be reduced, and she would be less depressed. I said, "Much of the loss that you have endured will have a lasting impact on your life, but your life is worth living for yourself and your children."

I also said that I knew the interview had been difficult—to remember these traumatic events. I emphasized that she might have more nightmares for a few nights but that these would diminish. I also mentioned that subsequent interviews would not be so difficult.

I started her on imipramine 50 mg (to be increased to 100 mg) at night and clonidine. I saw her individually with an interpreter every few weeks, and she attended a Cambodian support group. She showed symptomatic improvement, with a very much improved mood and an almost absence of nightmares in the 3 years that she was in treatment.

This interview took place several years ago, but I remember vividly how I felt. It was a draining experience with sadness for her and what she had endured. I did feel I had made a connection with her. I was less concerned about suicide, partly because completed suicide is rare among Cambodians, and in our experience it has been almost nonexistent. Also, the patient made a personal nonsuicide agreement with me.

I spent some time after the interview debriefing with my mental health counselor, Ben, who as a Cambodian himself often had more personal reactions to the patient's history. We discussed this patient and how she would likely do in the future. There is probably much more we should have processed, but it was time then for the next patient. The clinic continued, and Ben and I proceeded with the next interview.

MAIN CLINICAL APPROACHES FOR DIAGNOSING REFUGEE PATIENTS

Interviewing refugee patients requires competent and sympathetic interpreters who translate the psychiatrist's words and medical information accurately and who also can provide relevant cultural information. The psychiatrist should not worry about minor cultural issues and concerns the patients may have about him or her. All patients, by the time they have seen a psychiatrist, have been interviewed by American doctors and know that doctors ask intrusive questions in order to help them. It is only when psychiatrists are not active in the medical model, are silent and provide little feedback, that the patients become confused. This is not a place for a passive approach. With medical interviewing, taking a history, making a diagnosis, and providing relevant information to the patient give the patient an understandable experience.

Initial interviewing by the psychiatrist requires a slow, gentle approach (Kinzie 1981). Refugee patients are often intimidated by doctors and may be ashamed by things that have happened to them in the past. An accepting nonconfrontive approach both provides the basis for trust and serves as an an opportunity for the patient to teach the psychiatrist about his or her culture.

The initial evaluation with refugees is very unusual, as compared with other psychiatric evaluations. Refugees' traumatic experiences are often of very cruel and inhumane events and are difficult both for the patient to relate and the psychiatrist to hear. The interview must not concentrate only on the traumas; it must also focus on the patient's life before and after the traumatic events, as well as the current stresses in United States. The traumatic stories are important not only to obtain information but also to demonstrate that the psychiatrist can tolerate the pain and not retreat into professional objectivity, nor become overinvolved with a loss of boundaries. Although the interview can easily lead to a diagnosis, the patient needs to receive an explanation rather than just hear a diagnosis. The patient needs to hear some statement or explanation that connects the symptoms and their lives into a coherent story.

In my experience, insomnia and nightmares, which those afflicted find frightening, and irritability are the most common symptoms reported by patients with PTSD. It is necessary to put the patient's in some perspective—that is, "You are a strong person, but you have had many very difficult experiences. These experiences affected your body and your mind and cause poor sleep and nightmares, and make you easily upset."

Following the interview and agreement with the patient about the most disturbing symptom, there should be a joint agreement on treatment—namely, a focus on symptom reduction with realism. "We cannot bring back your country or your family or your friends who have been lost, but with medicine and talking about your current situation, we can help you sleep better, have fewer nightmares, and have less anger." When the depressive symptoms and PTSD symptoms have been reduced, supportive psychotherapy usually deals well with the day-to-day problems of a refugee. Helping with these everyday problems usually has priority over talking about the past traumatic experiences. The everyday problems of refugees include experiencing loneliness, learning English, finding a job, coping with children who are learning a different culture, and dealing with marital conflicts. Being confronted daily with these problems, which are often extremely difficult to resolve, adds to the stress of adjusting to a new country.

Severe PTSD for most refugee patients is a chronic disorder with remissions and exacerbations. There will be ups and downs. Reactivation, usually due to triggers of trauma such as news of fighting in the patient's own country, an auto accident, a severe illness, or the death of a friend, can occur after a long period of remission.

There is no expectation of a termination. We give refugee patients the paradoxical advice: "You will get better, *and* you can stay in a program as long as you need to." Many patients continue in the program past the time they have no active symptoms. On the other hand, many patients do leave and then return to our program when their symptoms recur. They are welcomed back.

Medical problems are very common among refugees. Many refugees have had very little medical care in the past. Diabetes and hypertension are very prevalent in the refugees, occurring at much higher rates than in the American population. These illnesses need to be continually evaluated in refugee patients in treatment. Most patients will have some medical insurance. A special group of refugees, asylum seekers, has no financial or medical support from the government during the time the asylum process is being evaluated. With federal grant funds allocated to treat torture victims, we have been able to provide some psychiatric help for the asylum seekers who are victims of torture. The psychiatrist, in the treatment of asylum seekers, has a dual role. He or she often is treating very traumatized asylum seekers and, at the same time, providing evidence to courts to help evaluate these patients' claims for asylum. Such court cases usually require clinical evidence indicating the experience of severe trauma, coupled with a current clear harm or danger to the person if he or she were to be deported back to the country of torture.

Working with refugees, especially those with severe trauma, can be emotionally draining, especially when the clinician is trying to help people whose lives have been disrupted with traumas and multiple losses. It can be overwhelming just hearing the stories when there is nothing to really "fix." The issue is often what to say when there is nothing to say. The most important issue for psychiatrists' health and their capacity to competently deliver care is to prevent the empathetic strain or countertransference that can occur related to the psychiatrist's frustration that "the system" will not provide enough help and/or to the psychiatrist's anger at the inexplicable cruelty that human beings bring to other human beings.

We psychiatrists need to take care of ourselves, both physically and emotionally. A type of support comes when one works with refugee patients over a long time and sees them improve, live productive lives, and hears them express their appreciation of our efforts. This phenomenon very importantly actually provides the necessary support and energy to keep us doing this work.

WHEN INTERVIEWING REFUGEES IS DONE POORLY

Psychiatric interviewing refugees is a difficult task, and many times it is done poorly, whether through inexperience, lack of time, or lack of the courage to face the terrible events.

A common problem is reliance on rating scales. Trauma and depression scales, if validated in the patient's own language, can provide some information about symptoms, but only for the disorders for which the scale was developed. There are other disorders, such as traumatic brain injury or psychosis, which will be missed. The trauma scale may register a specific trauma, such as rape, but the scale does not reveal how and when. Was it one time? Was it a gang rape? Did it occur while the husband was being killed? In other words, the scales cannot put the events in a context or in a chronological order with other events or symptoms.

Example

A man from a West African country sought asylum in the United States because of persecution from the government. He had belonged to an opposition political party and had been tortured, and he had symptoms of PTSD. When asked further about this, he related a story of having suffered child abuse by a relative, which was the source of his symptoms.

A second problem is to lightly pass over or not inquire further about the traumatic events. "It was awful, with people dying" is a statement that should not pass. Sometimes psychiatrists and patients passively agree not to discuss or talk about these events. An opportunity is then missed to gently push for information or to ask about feelings (i.e., "How did it feel to see suffering and death around you?"). This is a chance for the patient to reflect on the events, and his or her own reactions, and personal pain. It is important for the psychiatrist to hear the stories, to show that he or she can tolerate the vicarious pain and quietly empathize with the patient.

A third problem is for the psychiatrist to take the history and respond in the "right way" but to not establish a real connection with the patient. "Sorry you have so many problems." This may be a standard psychiatric response, but given in a detached manner it does not help connect the psychiatrist with the patient. Empathy is what the patient needs, and its absence is felt by the patient.

It is difficult to describe an empathetic relationship, but for the psychiatrist to be engaged nonverbally with a body language with attention on the patient is clearly a start. There is often nothing to say, and quietness indicates taking the information in and allows the patient to go on. When the psychiatrist feels the connection, there is real sharing and deepening of the interview.

The goal of the interview is not just to get information but also to establish a relationship that can provide safety for long-term treatment and drug treatment.

CODA

The patient returned to the clinic, 14 years after her last visit, with a complaint of being "sick too much." She described poor sleep, sleeping only 2–3 hours a night, interrupted by nightmares. During the 14 years since her last clinic visit, she had been able to work and had been involved in a sustained relationship. However, a few months prior to her coming back to the clinic, she received from her sister a picture of her father that she had never seen before.

The picture brought back to her memory something she had suppressed—the death of her father. She was beside her father, with her sister, as the father was tied up, his abdomen cut open, and his liver cut out. Since receiving the picture of her father, the patient had had many recurrent nightmares and intrusive memories of her father being killed. She also had experienced irritability, startle reaction, and many thoughts of suicide. She told the story in a hesitant manner, crying profusely in the interview as she recounted events that had occurred 25 years previously.

It was a case of reactivation of the symptoms. However, this actual experience was much more than that. The patient was getting in touch with a severe traumatic event, which she had barely mentioned before to anyone and had suppressed much of her life. The patient and I went through the same previous discussion that we had had about agreement of the goals of treatment at the beginning of her psychiatric care in our clinic.

With treatment, medicine, and the support of a group of Cambodian patients, this patient improved. She continued in treatment for 3 more years.

KEY CLINICAL POINTS

- The diagnostic interview of refugee psychiatric patients is difficult, requiring a gentle, slow approach to promote trust and set the relationship for long-term care.

- An interpreter who knows the culture and language of the patient and is correctly interpreting the patient's affect as well as content is essential.

- The interview format includes the present/primary complaint, which is usually psychological symptoms, and a chronological social and developmental history, including life before the traumatic events. The psychiatrist should have a general idea of the severe problems in the patient's country, including war, government persecution and torture, and starvation conditions, and the time frame within which these problems occurred.

- The traumatic events specific to the patient need to be covered as completely as the patient's comfort allows. These include very traumatic events, death of family, personal persecution and torture, unwanted sexual attacks, long-term trauma, starvation, and diseases. It is important to ask about the patient's feelings and about these events.

- Although it may be difficult to discuss, traumatic events from life in the refugee camp and life in the United States need to be addressed.
- A mental status examination is necessary, because psychotic or organic brain disorders may be present.
- At the end of the interview, the psychiatrist should summarize what he or she heard and clarify with the patient the goals of treatment.
- The psychiatrist should be hopeful but realistic, with clear expectations of treatment and reduction of symptoms, including depressive symptoms, as the goal.

REFERENCES

The History Place: Genocide in the 20th century: Pol Pot in Cambodia 1975–1979. 2,000,000 deaths. 1999 Available at: http://www.historyplace.com/worldhistory/genocide/pol-pot.htm. Accessed October 23, 2019.

Kinzie JD: Evaluation and psychotherapy of Indochinese refugee patients. Am J Psychother 35(2):251–261, 1981 7258422

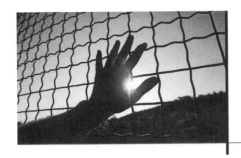

Chapter 3

PSYCHOLOGICAL TREATMENT

Narrative Exposure Therapy

Linda Piwowarczyk, M.D., M.P.H.
Dhanviney Verma, M.D.

CONSIDERATIONS WHEN DOING THERAPY WITH REFUGEE POPULATIONS

As was highlighted in Chapter 1, the rise in complex humanitarian disasters globally has resulted in unprecedented numbers of displaced persons around the world. People have been known to flee outright conflict, threats of violence and sexual violence, ethnic cleansing, the strategic use of rape during conflict, family loss, torture, persecution, lack of safety in refugee camps when gathering firewood, and extreme hardship. As such, traumatic events can occur in the country of origin, leading to refugee flows, and during transit, as well as in the country of resettlement. We have become all too familiar through media with the overloaded leaderless boats traversing the Mediterranean, having lost some of their occupants, which evokes memories of those fleeing by boat from Vietnam while fighting pirates in their path; those walking amid landmines fleeing their homes; or the young boys and girls from Sudan crisscrossing the country heading to Kenya. These are the stories that people carry with them as they come to our clinics, hospitals, and emergency rooms. Notwithstanding what people have gone through, increasing attention is being paid toward the mental health impact of postmigration stressors across varied displaced populations. A briefing paper, "Trauma and Mental Health in Forcibly Displaced Populations," available from the International Society for Traumatic Stress Studies, reminds us that these stressors can be grouped into three general categories: social isolation and discrimination, socioeconomic factors, and immigration and refugee policies (Nickerson et al. 2017). These are important points for providers across all disciplines, more so in behavioral health, to consider while providing competent care to this population.

From a mental health standpoint, recognizing the cultural barriers of our patients in seeking services is crucial to successful psychotherapeutic intervention. As Derr and colleagues (2016) note, such barriers most often include stigma and beliefs or norms about mental illness followed by preference for alternative services, language, distrust of formal providers, self or family reliance, and acculturation difficulties. The social deterrents of health affecting this population include language, high cost, lack of knowledge of resources, transportation problems/inaccessibility, lack of insurance, lack of documentation and fear of deportation proceeded by long wait, provider culture incompetence, fear of missing work, lack of collaboration between services and churches, general structural barriers, competing health demands, gender of provider, and discrimination (Derr et al. 2016).

IMPACT OF TRAUMA

In a study of more than 3,000 respondents from postconflict communities in Algeria, Cambodia, Ethiopia, and Palestine, there were differential responses to violence, with varying rates of PTSD, mood disorders, anxiety disorders, and somatoform disorders depending on the country (de Jong et al. 2003). In another study of 854 war refugees from the former Yugoslavia living in Germany, Italy, and the United Kingdom (≥ 255 per country), although the prevalence rates of mental disorders varied substantially across the three countries, a number of associations did not. A lower level of education, more traumatic experiences during and after the war, more migration-related stress, a temporary residence permit, and not feeling accepted were independently associated with higher rates of mood and anxiety disorders. Mood disorders were also associated with older age, female gender, and being unemployed, and anxiety disorders with the absence of combat experience. Older age, a lower level of education, more traumatic experiences during and after the war, absence of combat experience, more migration-related stress, and a temporary residence permit predisposed one to PTSD. Of note, substance use disorders were associated with younger age, male gender, and not living with a partner. As noted above, the associations did not differ significantly across the countries (Bogic et al. 2012). In a meta-analysis of 181 studies representing 81,866 refugees and other conflicted persons from 40 countries, being a torture survivor was the strongest factor associated with PTSD (OR=2.01) followed by cumulative exposure to other potentially traumatic events (OR=1.52), time since conflict (OR=0.77), and assessed level of political terror (OR=1.60). Depression was associated with other potentially traumatic events (OR=1.64), time since conflict (OR=0.80), reported torture (OR=1.48), and residency status (OR = 1.30) (Steel et al. 2009).

From the standpoint of psychiatric morbidity, in a cohort of 9,025 patients treated by members of the National Consortium of Torture Treatment Programs in the United States, 69% of survivors studied had PTSD, 52.4% had major depressive disorder, and 35% had comorbid PTSD and major depressive disorder (Member Centers of the National Consortium of Torture Treatment Programs [NCTTP] 2015). Further study of torture survivors has underscored the importance of getting people into treatment, because time spent before presenting for services was found to significantly predict anxiety, PTSD, and depression. Moreover, cumulative exposure to multiple torture types predicted anxiety and PTSD, whereas mental health, basic resources (access to food, shelter, medical care), and external risks (risk of being victimized at home, community, work, or school) were the strongest psychosocial predictors of anxiety, PTSD, and depression—findings that also have implications for treatment (Song et al. 2018).

ELEMENTS OF A THOUGHTFUL INTERVIEW

When asked what was the biggest concern when first coming to our program in Boston, a patient replied: "I did not know how I would be received." We have learned through our work the importance of meeting people where they are at and addressing them from a multidisciplinary perspective that we have come to refer to as our own version of radical hospitality. Working from this perspective is coupled with having a patient-centered approach. Our intake is a "bio-psycho-social-spiritual" assessment. The assessment is coupled with meeting a patient navigator who orients the new patient both to our program and hospital and to the U.S. health care system overall. The visit is completed when the patient is referred to the food pantry located at the hospital, appointments are set up at various clinics as needed, and information is given regarding local legal services. This initial meeting does involve getting elements of one's trauma story, which is reflective of one's own worldview and understanding of causes based on one's worldview, as well as expectations. Asking about the historical context of the patient's suffering often provides a more meaningful substrate for therapy and also helps with alliance building. For some, although it is difficult at times to find the words to express one's sorrow or experiences of betrayal and suffering, the opportunity to speak and be listened to often provides some relief. For others, being provided a space where one can cry freely is what is needed. By creating a treatment plan, there is the opportunity for the enhancement of self-agency, which is critical, especially when one has been in forced situations absent free will. Meeting people where they are at becomes a foundation to establishing hope and a sense of security.

A health professional may be the first person to whom one discloses what one has experienced. Authorities who should be protecting the civilian population are often the culprits, or in the case of ethnic cleansing perpetrators at times are members of the community or even neighbors. It is in the relationship between the torturer and the one tortured that the profound fracture in trust occurs. As such, it is also in the relationship between survivor and healer and the institution in which one works that the restoration of human connection can begin to take place. It is crucial how one is received by a program. Creating a sense of safety is central to this work. Understanding what the survivor may have experienced, and the conditions, cultural practices, and health beliefs in the country and region of origin, are all significant to helping him or her feel understood. The necessity to leave one's homeland and being forced into exile, as well as the intentionality of torture, has a grave impact on human dignity.

Often refugees do not make the connection between their symptoms and their traumatic experiences. One goal is to avoid retraumatizing the patient during the clinical encounter. How one experiences events will often influence if they are viewed as traumatic. There is much variability in how people express reactions to traumatic stress. Understanding trauma through a broader lens helps one to appreciate the sociocultural and political context. As inquiries are made, the clinician must be sensitized toward not triggering the patient. He or she must be mindful, for example, not to simulate an interrogation. Providing psychoeducation about trauma and traumatic reactions, teaching grounding techniques, and ensuring safety in the environment are foundational. Using a strengths perspective and connecting to the pretrauma self are important. Being mindful how one can establish social connections is important—here communities of faith may have great importance, as refugees often come from collectivist cultures. Being mindful of the need to pace is essential—take breaks and avoid overwhelming the patient. "What would make you comfortable?" is often a good inquiry when the clinician is attempting to build rapport at the initial visit and when he or she notices signs of distress.

There may be a reluctance to ask about torture. One can say, "The people from your country or in your situation have sometimes experienced torture. Has that ever happened to you? Or "It is not uncommon for people in captivity to be harmed by police, military, or security operatives. Has that ever happen to you?" Being knowledgeable about where someone comes from and what is happening in that country can be very useful, as can a basic understanding of rules governing immigration. Stabilization and establishment of trust are critical. A chronological perspective can be helpful to understanding one's experience. The clinician must first understand why someone left his or her country and what he or she experienced "preflight." There may be one traumatic event or a series of events that leads someone to leave his or her country. This may involve conflict, arrests, involvement in demonstrations, betrayal. It is a significant decision to decide to flee leaving all that one knows behind, without necessarily the prospects of returning. This is perhaps best summarized by the word "loss." It is also important to understand the ways in which one was successful in one's country of origin. During flight, crossing a border is often fraught with danger and much uncertainty. This process can take place over an extended period of time and may involve periods of having to hide. One can be met by violence, exploitation, or even land mines. Finally, postflight may mean arrival in a safer environment, adjustment to a new country or culture, poverty, discrimination, and pressure to be self-sufficient, and legal hurdles can challenge one's original expectations.

Work with uprooted populations can often require the need for professional interpreters, some of whom have had their own experiences of refugee trauma or torture. That said, it is helpful to talk with the interpreter before and after the clinical encounter. Seating should be set up in such a way that the clinician is speaking slowly and directly to the patient or client. It is best when simple language is used and there are sufficient pauses. It is necessary to allow the interpreter to finish interpreting before asking the next question. The clinician should avoid the use of slang. Procedures should be explained step by step. The clinician should also confirm that the client understands. The client should not be left alone with the interpreter. The interpreter should not be requested to perform functions outside of his or her role. In-person interpreting rather than telephonic is preferred, especially when, for example, clients or patients are confused or impaired, angry or upset, have speech or hearing problems or head injuries, are traumatized, or are small children (Bancroft 2014).

BRIEF LITERATURE REVIEW OF PSYCHOTHERAPY WITH REFUGEES AND ASYLUM SEEKERS

Given that PTSD with comorbid mood disorders remains the most prevalent condition among refugees and asylum seekers, most research has focused on improvement in trauma symptomatology as an indicator of intervention efficacy. In McFarlane and Kaplan's (2012) review of a mix of 40 randomized controlled trials (RCTs), nonrandomized trials, and single-cohort follow-up studies, conducted over a 30-year period, that investigated interventions for adult survivors of torture and trauma, about 90% of the studies demonstrated significant improvements on at on at least one outcome measure related to posttraumatic stress, depression, anxiety, and somatic symptoms. However, it should be noted that little evidence was available regarding the effect on treatment outcomes of the amount, type, or length of treatment; the influence of patient characteristics; maintenance of treatment effects; and treatment outcomes other than psychiatric symptomatology. The first Cochrane review that aimed to assess the beneficial and adverse effects of psychological, social, and welfare interventions for torture survivors was published in 2014 (Patel et al. 2014) and included nine RCTs from European and African countries in the meta-analysis. Patel et al. (2014) reported that all trials provided psychological interventions only, with no immediate benefits observed on posttraumatic symptoms, distress, or quality of life. However, moderate benefits with small sample size were demonstrated for narrative exposure therapy (NET) and cognitive-behavioral therapy (CBT) in reducing distress and PTSD at a 6-month follow-up, although the evidence was of very low quality. Inherent in the nature of research pertaining to this topic, the review authors commented on various gaps, including a lack of culturally appropriate psychometric measures free from biases that would also correlate symptom reduction with improved quality of life and participation in the community. However, a more recent review by Tribe et al. (2017) reported positive outcomes from NET in refugees from a diverse range of backgrounds and trauma types, and less evidence for standard CBT and eye movement desensitization and reprocessing (EMDR)—approaches that are indicated in the general population with PTSD.

NET is a short-term manualized treatment that is

> a form of exposure that encourages traumatized survivors to tell their detailed life history chronologically to a skilled counselor or psychotherapist who will record it, read it back, and assist the survivor with the task of integrating fragmented traumatic memories into a coherent narrative....Originally developed for survivors of multiple and complex forms of trauma who come from diverse backgrounds and who live in unsafe situations, often under conditions of continuous trauma, narrative exposure serves not only therapeutic purposes but also a social and political agenda. While NET is treating survivors through the narrative process, it is also simultaneously documenting violations of child rights and human rights. (Schauer et al. 2011, p. 3)

As summarized by Lely et al. (2019), NET is a

> standardized form of TF [trauma-focused] psychotherapy, embedding trauma exposure in an autobiographical context. The manual recommends 4–12 sessions of 90 minutes' duration, depending on the number of traumatic events (Schauer et al. 2011), and treatment focuses on imaginary trauma exposure and on reorganizing memories (Schnyder et al. 2015). Memories of traumatic events are hypothesized to form multiple fear networks dominated by sensory-perceptual information and lacking autobiographical information (Schauer et al. 2011). By connecting these anxiety-provoking implicit memories with episodic context, the autobiographic memory is rebuilt, allowing for reduction of anxiety (Schauer et al. 2011). In NET, the therapist and the patient create a timeline of the patient's life, followed by chronologically elaborating this timeline in subsequent sessions. At the end of therapy, the patient receives the written narrative as a documented testimony. Given its focus on the lifespan, NET is particularly suited to populations affected by multiple traumatic experiences. (Schauer et al. 2011)

The European Association for Psychotherapy (EAP), in its guidelines related to work with refugees, recognized that issues related to safety and to separation from family members and their possibly uncertain fate often must be addressed before one can address the processing of trauma. EAP also cautions its members to be aware of differences in cultural backgrounds from self, to update their knowledge and reassess their beliefs and practices, and to be aware of the risk of secondary trauma, vicarious traumatization, and burnout in themselves and the interpreters with whom they work, for whom EAP also recommends special training. Using the Istanbul Protocol, EAP urges, with client permission, that psychotherapists properly document sequelae to crime and human rights violations, and also write a report on such evidence if requested by the client or to secure documentation by an outside expert (European Association for Psychotherapy 2017). "Culture in the context of these guidelines is understood to include religious, ethnic, language and social factors, political background and group identities that shape refugees and their core identities in a varying degree" (European Association for Psychotherapy 2017, p. 4).

DOING PSYCHOTHERAPY

From our collective experience, we highlight below the broader concepts of stigma, cultural humility, and vicarious traumatization with critical therapy topics rooted in identity crisis (collective and individual) and loss of self and life purpose through case examples.

STIGMA

As has been summarized by Carpenter-Song et al. (2010), culture has an impact on the identification and definition of illnesses and their meaningfulness, the variance with respect to timing and onset, presenting symptoms, course, outcome treatment utilization, and responses (Carpenter-Song et al. 2010). Our clinic experience is similar to fieldwork with Congolese and Somali communities showing that mental health concerns in these communities are principally associated with more extreme situations in which erratic or noticeable behaviors are present. There is significant stigma in the community related to both having a mental health problem and seeking treatment. The frame of reference for intervention is generally the country of origin. As a result, there is a greater proclivity to turn to family or friends for support, to use traditional ways of healing in coping with stress and depression, or to turn to religion. Mental health services and mental health needs from a Western perspective are not understood in these communities. The actual role of mental health professionals, especially psychiatrists, is also not understood, nor is it clear to these communities what symptoms can be treated. Moreover, there is much ambivalence about the use of medication. In addition, the idea of talking to a stranger, someone not from the culture, is generally frowned upon (Piwowarczyk et al. 2014).

Case 1

Mirembe, a 34-year-old Nigerian woman, had been brutally raped by multiple men while detained for allegedly spreading HIV due to her homosexual orientation. She suffered from chronic low self-esteem rooted in rejection by her family and community. The socially expected identity was something that was to be learned, and any accompanying psychological distress was to be addressed by family, and not outsiders, including therapists, since especially in her case that would bring shame to her family if her community were to become aware of her struggles. Her early adulthood was marred by an abusive husband from a forced marriage. Moreover, she was also blamed for her mother's death.

Mirembe entered weekly therapy for twelve 90-minute sessions with much reluctance because she was fearful of being seen as "crazy," which might isolate her from her new community postmigration; not being believed by anyone, including her providers; being hospitalized if she disclosed anything about her suicidal ideations; experiencing retraumatization while narrating; and experiencing long-standing shame and feelings of helplessness contributing to poor understanding of the role of mental health professionals.

The first two sessions were spent on conducting diagnostic interview and providing psychoeducation about the diagnosis of PTSD. A brief neurobiological underpinning of the fear network was discussed in relation to the specific role and the format of NET. During the next session, the therapist gently constructed an overview of her life story without getting details of the "hot memories" that invoked sensory, cognitive, and emotional distress. These first few sessions were vital in establishing a therapeutic alliance and building trust.

It is worth noting that the action to bear witness to their suffering—which is by no means an easy task, and a patient can certainly test a therapist's capability to engage in such an interaction before even disclosing any information—holds therapeutic value in itself. As such, it is important for a therapist to not simulate the victim-aggressor dynamic in the session and to listen with cultural curiosity and explore the patient's traumatic experiences when the patient's "ego" has regained sufficient consistency to rewitness the experience (Luci 2017). The initial phase in therapy, besides addressing the acculturation and postmigration stressors to restore some sense of cohesion, therefore includes the evaluation of a patient's inner psychological constructs.

Case 1 (*continued*)

In the subsequent eight sessions, Mirembe narrated her struggles, which were fragmented by the intrusive memories of the multiple events that had been placed on the timeline constructed earlier. The therapist helped her face the psychological discomfort through imaginal exposure and sensations of hyperarousal symptoms while reframing her experiences in a meaningful context. She was invited to review after each trauma to add to or correct the narrative. During the last session, the therapist read the full integrated narrative and provided her with a typed copy.

With time, in a safe, nonjudgmental, empathic holding environment, Mirembe was able to explore her prior experiences to integrate her fragmented sense of self to optimize her coping strengths and find a new occupation. This experience provided her with an opportunity to speak up and expand her voice in a trusting stable relationship, an experience that was foreign to her. The treatment course, culminating in a visual testimony of her suffering while bridging the disconnected emotional circuitry, began the internal process of healing and regaining her dignity.

CULTURAL HUMILITY

Within global health settings there has been an evolution from the concept of cultural sensitivity (approaching individuals with health beliefs different from those of providers) to cultural competence (interacting effectively with people of difference cultures) to cultural humility (undergoing a continual, lifelong process of self-reflection and self-critique that overtly addresses the power inequities between providers and clients, rather than mastering a culture) (Miller 2009). In an effort to summarize cultural humility by meta-analysis, a series of attributes have been identified by Foronda et al. (2016): namely, openness (an open mind; willingness to explore new ideas when interacting with a culturally diverse individual); self-awareness (awareness of one's strengths, limitations, values, beliefs, behavior, and appearance to others); egolessness (humbleness); supportive interaction (intersections of existence among individuals leading to positive human exchanges); and self-reflection and critique (reflecting on one's thoughts, feelings, and actions). The authors point out that cultural humility means being aware of power imbalances and "being humble in every interaction with every individual" (Foronda et al. 2016).

Case 2

Mariyo, a mother of five, never attended school and had an arranged marriage. The rebels who were in control of the area detained and attacked the family, because of the family's ethnicity, in their home in

Mogadishu. They killed her husband in front of the family. She and her children fled. On route, one son was killed and a daughter died from starvation. When she originally presented with symptoms of major depression and PTSD, she was treated with sertraline and individual treatment, which involved processing her trauma experiences in her country of origin and in flight. She later joined a women's group, which she found very helpful as a support to adjusting to life in the United States. She obtained U.S. citizenship.

She presented to her former psychiatrist some years later with insomnia of approximately 1 month's duration that coincided with a recent move with her son and his family to the first floor of a nearby apartment complex. She presented with dizziness and lack of sleep—only sleeping a few nights a week. Before moving into the new apartment, she had religious leaders from the community come to bless the apartment. She no longer felt depressed. Her energy was reduced, and she attributed this to her age. Her sleep was reduced and interrupted, but she could not quantify the length of time she would actually sleep. She had persistent concentration and memory problems that were not progressive. Her appetite was normal. She had many friends in both the new and old buildings with whom she kept in contact by phone and in person. She denied any nightmares or flashbacks. She was not afraid but preferred not to go out at night alone. She avoided crowds as well as talking with people who spoke about the ongoing violence in their homeland. She was not irritable, nor did she feel numb. She recalled the main events that had happened to her. She was not sure if she could live a long life because she felt that the Angel of Death was about. In the new building, there were noises. She decided that they were a result of spirits called *jinn* in her home, but she did not specifically think that the jinn wanted to hurt her. She believed that the jinn were indirectly related to her insomnia. The solution to the problem was twofold. She planned to talk with spiritual leaders in the community to perform a special ceremony involving Koranic verses in her home to eradicate the jinn, while at the same time consenting to the use of melatonin to address her insomnia. It was necessary to allow for broader cultural and spiritual understanding of the problem while at the same time holding a Western approach.

VICARIOUS TRAUMATIZATION

Working with uprooted populations can be very challenging in part related to the extent of trauma and, in many cases, betrayal. Our patients often face deep existential issues. We as clinicians are brought into the clinical space of hearing examples of grave cruelty and suffering. Our patients often turn to us to carry their hope. It is necessary for us to confront our own thoughts about the presence of evil in the world. It is important in doing this work to be attentive to its impact on our lives. Working in a trauma-informed environment is required. Being able to share with colleagues our countertransference responses is a necessary part of the work. Prioritizing self-care is not a luxury but rather a necessity. This work highlights the polarity of the human experience: from the depths of cruelty that human beings are capable of inflicting on one another to the heights of the profound dignity of the human spirit. The latter is often the inspiration behind the work. As health professionals, we bear witness to these extreme realities. Being fully present to the work in the room is essential.

Vicarious traumatization is defined by Pearlman and Saakvitne (1995) as "a transformation in one's inner experience resulting from empathic engagement with clients' traumatic material." Secondary traumatic stress symptoms can also result from hearing traumatic material but tends to be more observable external symptoms than vicarious traumatization (Pearlman and Saakvitne 1995, p. 151). A newer concept, *vicarious resilience*, refers to unique, positive effects that transform therapists in response to witnessing trauma survivors' resilience and recovery process (Killian et al. 2017). Preventive factors that should be under consideration include such things as attending to self-care, having solid professional training in psychotherapy, fostering therapeutic self-awareness, participating in regular self-examination by collegial and external supervision, limiting caseload, and keeping a balance between empathy and proper distance to clients (Pross 2006).

SOME THOUGHTS ABOUT GROUP THERAPY

Kira et al. (2012) point out the importance of group therapy to address not only past trauma and present stresses (taking into account potential individual pathology) but also traumas related to their collective identities and cumulative trauma given the role of collectivist cultures in which healing often takes place within a group context. That said, empirical literature is limited with respect to group work. Kira et al. (2012) summarize several types of group work with refugees and torture survivors—namely, integrated models of combined individual and group therapy, time-limited groups, and multiple family groups—as well as nontraditional activity groups. They further note that homogeneity by gender has advantages in cultural, religious, and clinical domains and allows ethnic pride to rise to the surface. Multiethnic groups that speak the same language aid in creating tolerance and adjustment to the U.S. multicultural society. Using the opportunity to address discrimination and oppression in groups is also an important activity (Kira et al. 2012).

Work with refugees and survivors of torture is often a long-standing process with bonds that transcend time. It is a profoundly humbling experience to accompany patients through their process of recovery, as we are witnesses both to the worst of humanity and to the strength of the human spirit. The work can be very challenging. However, to see people love again and establish community and thrive inspires providers to embrace this work. Cases are often left open, in that after the original work is done, it is not uncommon for patients to reconnect during times of crisis and uncertainty. Our experience also suggests that at times of joy or significant milestones, our patients wish to share their accomplishments from job and educational successes, family reunifications, or concerns about immigration or insurance. Unlike in a Western context, we care providers often come to be viewed as family or elders.

KEY CLINICAL POINTS

- Recognizing cultural barriers, such as stigmatization or fear of mental illness, on the part of refugees seeking services is critical for effective and accurate therapeutic intervention by the psychiatrist.

- Cultural humility, characterized by openness, self-awareness, humbleness, and reflecting on one's thoughts, feelings, and actions, is an important therapist attribute for treating refugees.

- Refugees are often reluctant to talk about trauma and torture. Furthermore, many refugees do not distinguish between symptoms and traumatic experiences.

- The therapeutic technique of using the patient's narrative within a stable treatment relationship with a therapist helps the patient be able to experience the psychological discomfort that may occur during the therapy.

- The patient's ability to develop a coherent chronological narrative allows the patient to reframe his or her role as a survivor.

- Narrative exposure therapy can greatly open the patient to some of the trauma experienced and put it into a chronological perspective of his or her life.

- Working with traumatized refuges can be a long process, and it is a profoundly humbling experience to accompany patients through this process of recovery.

REFERENCES

Bancroft MA: Cultural Competence: A Trainer's Guide. Columbia, MD, Culture and Language Press, 2014

Bogic M, Ajdukovic D, Bremner S, et al: Factors associated with mental disorders in long-settled war refugees: refugees from the former Yugoslavia in Germany, Italy and the UK. Br J Psychiatry 200(3):216–223, 2012 22282430

Carpenter-Song E, Chu E, Drake RE, et al: Ethno-cultural variations in the experience and meaning of mental illness and treatment: implications for access and utilization. Transcult Psychiatry 47(2):224–251, 2010 20603387

de Jong JT, Komproe IH, Van Ommeren M: Common mental disorders in postconflict settings. Lancet 361(9375):2128–2130, 2003 12826440

Derr AS: Mental health service use among immigrants in the United States: a systematic review. Psychiatr Serv 67(3):265–274, 2016 26695493

European Association for Psychotherapy: European Association for Psychotherapy (EAP) position statement and specific guidelines: psychotherapy with refugees— Task force for this position statement and guidelines: members and consultants. March 29, 2017. Available at: https://www.europsyche.org/app/uploads/2019/05/EAP-Guidelines-Psychotherapy-with-Refugees_final-officia.pdf. Accessed October 8, 2019.

Foronda C, Baptiste DL, Reinholdt MM, et al: Cultural humility: a concept analysis. J Transcult Nurs 27(3):210–217, 2016 26122618

Killian K, Hernandez-Wolfe P, Engstrom D, et al: Development of the Vicarious Resilience Scale (VRS): a measure of positive effects of working with trauma survivors. Psychol Trauma 9(1):23–31, 2017 27710002

Kira IA, Ahmed A, Wasim F, et al: Group therapy for refugees and torture survivors: treatment model innovations. Int J Group Psychother 62(1):69–88, 2012 22229369

Lely JCG, Smid GE, Jongedijk RA, et al: The effectiveness of narrative exposure therapy: a review, meta-analysis and meta-regression analysis. Eur J Psychotraumatol 10(1):1550344, 2019 31007868

Luci M: Disintegration of the self and the regeneration of "psychic skin" in the treatment of traumatized refugees. J Anal Psychol 62(2):227–246, 2017 28321873

McFarlane CA, Kaplan I: Evidence-based psychological interventions for adult survivors of torture and trauma: a 30-year review. Transcult Psychiatry 49(3–4):539–567, 2012 23008355

Member Centers of the National Consortium of Torture Treatment Programs (NCTTP): Descriptive, inferential, functional outcome data on 9,025 torture survivors over six years in the United States. Torture 25(2):34–60, 2015 26932129

Miller S: Cultural humility is the first step to becoming global care providers. J Obstet Gynecol Neonatal Nurs 38(1):92–93, 2009 19208053

Nickerson A, Liddell B, Asnaani A, et al: Trauma and Mental Health in Forcibly Displaced Populations. Oakbrook Terrace, IL, International Society for Traumatic Stress Studies, 2017. Available at: http://www.istss.org/education-research/trauma-and-mental-health-in-forcibly-displaced-pop.aspx. Accessed October 24, 2019.

Patel N, Kellezi B, Williams AC: Psychological, social and welfare interventions for psychological health and well-being of torture survivors. Cochrane Database Syst Rev 11(11):CD009317, 2014 25386846

Pearlman LA, Saakvitne KW: Trauma and the Therapist: Counter Transference and Vicarious Traumatization in Psychotherapy With Incest Survivors. New York, WW Norton, 1995

Piwowarczyk L, Bishop H, Yusuf A, et al: Congolese and Somali beliefs about mental health services. J Nerv Ment Dis 202(3):209–216, 2014 24566506

Pross C: Burnout, vicarious traumatization and its prevention. Torture 16(1):1–9, 2006 17460342

Schauer M, Neumer F, Elbert T: Narrative Exposure Therapy: A Short Term Treatment for Traumatic Stress Disorders, 2nd Edition. Göttingen, Germany, Hogrefe & Huber, 2011

Schnyder U, Ehlers A, Elbert T, et al: Psychotherapies for PTSD: what do they have in common? Eur J Psychotraumatol 6:28186, 2015 26290178

Song SJ, Subica A, Kaplan C, et al: Predicting the mental health and functioning of torture survivors. J Nerv Ment Dis 206(1):33–39, 2018 28350563

Steel Z, Chey T, Silove D, et al: Association of torture and other potentially traumatic events with mental health outcomes among populations exposed to mass conflict and displacement: a systematic review and meta-analysis. JAMA 302(5):537–549, 2009 19654388

Tribe RH, Sendt KV, Tracy DK: A systematic review of psychosocial interventions for adult refugees and asylum seekers. J Mental Health May 9:1–15, 2017 28485636

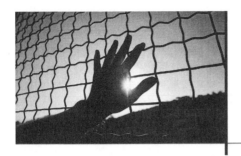

Chapter 4

PSYCHOTHERAPY FOR
POSTMIGRATION STRESS

J. David Kinzie, M.D., FACPsych, DLFAPA

Refugees usually have experienced severe trauma, and as a result, about 80% in our patient population have PTSD. There is now much empirical data about the treatment of PTSD. Evidence-based treatment has emphasized trauma-focused therapy as a first treatment, with cognitive processing and prolonged exposure also being supported (Charney et al. 2018). Refugees represent an unusual population, having multiple traumas. They also face issues of loss, including death of family members, and adjustment to new cultures and language, which causes new stress. Nevertheless, there are now suggestions about psychological treatment for refugees with PTSD. One review of treatments for psychological treatment of refugees found that trauma-focused therapy treatments have some efficacy (Nickerson et al. 2011). A more recent review also found more evidence for trauma-focused treatment, including eye movement desensitization and reprocessing and narrative exposure therapy, for refugees (Thompson et al. 2018; see also Chapter 3). However, these reviews miss several issues related to refugees. There is a high rate of co-morbidity between PTSD and depression. About half in one sample (Nickerson et al. 2017) had PTSD and major depression, and this comorbidity is present in about 80% of the patients in our own clinic. Comorbidity is associated with increased impairment burden (Nickerson et al. 2017) and complicates treatment. Refugees after resettlement also often experience new trauma or stressful events, and this increases or exacerbates recent symptoms (Schoch et al. 2016). Postmigration factors were found to impact 39% of treatment sessions in one study; these stresses included work-related issues, finances, and problems in family life (Bruhn et al. 2018).

PSYCHIATRIC TREATMENT FOR REFUGEES: INTERCULTURAL PSYCHIATRIC PROGRAM

The Intercultural Psychiatric Program began treating traumatized refugees even before DSM-III formulated the diagnosis of PTSD in 1980. Our approach was empirical and multimodal. The psychiatrist provided psychotherapy and medication for symptoms, and the ethnic mental health counselors provided consistent interpretation with support and education for patients. Later, the counselors facilitated support groups for their patients (see Chapter 6). Thus, the psychotherapeutic approach was always facilitated by mental health counselors who acted as interpreters and sometime cultural educators in all the sessions.

The original evaluation included a detailed symptom and social history, including all recounted traumas. This recounting was often very painful for our patients, and also difficult to hear, but it was necessary to let patients know we understood some of what they had been through. However, we did not, and do not, have a trauma-focused approach. The practical reason for this decision was that ongoing postmigration stresses—family conflict, raising children in a new culture, lack of income, lack of housing, and even everyday prejudice, including violence—were dominating the patients' lives. At that time, studies showing that non-trauma-focused therapy can be effective were not available. Our approach was very similar to interpersonal psychotherapy (IPT), which deals with interpersonal losses, role transitions, interpersonal conflict, and personal deficits. A randomized clinical trial for PTSD found IPT to be "non-inferior" to trauma-focused therapy sessions (Markowitz et al. 2015). Like our approach, IPT is practical and compatible with medicine and fits in with the supportive psychotherapy that psychiatrists traditionally do.

POSTMIGRATION FACTORS IN THERAPY

The following case illustrates that for a patient with existing PTSD, ongoing stress becomes the focus of therapy.

Case 1

The patient is a 47-year-old woman from Somalia. She came in because of multiple symptoms of depression, nightmares, startle reaction, and intrusive thoughts. She had a very abusive childhood: both of her parents died when she was young, and she was raised by an uncle and a cousin, both of whom were abusive toward her. Her first marriage resulted in seven pregnancies and five live children. Her husband never supported her and eventually took two more wives. In 1990 when the war broke out, gangs came into their neighborhood. When gang members charged into her house, she and the children were able to run away, but her two younger brothers were both murdered. Another time a gang challenged her and other women, and she barely got away without being raped. She spent 6 years in a refugee camp and came to the United States after that.

Her course over the next 17 years has been erratic. Personally, she has had multiple medical problems, including anemia, hypertension, osteoarthritis, poor hearing, and prediabetes. Her primary concerns during her psychotherapy for these years were her children. Two daughters have schizophrenia: one moved away, and one had been in and out of the hospital with marked agitation and aggressive behavior. A son dropped out of school, was charged with rape, and later used drugs and was gambling. She became very obsessed about her children's problems and never discussed past traumas. After a few years of treatment, she developed frank hallucinations and paranoia, which were more or less successfully treated with antipsychotics, but treatment was often interrupted with her nonattendance.

She seemed at times so preoccupied and overwhelmed by her children's problems she appeared to have early dementia, although her dementia-like symptoms cleared when the stress was reduced. She needed help getting to the office because she could not use transportation on her own. She also needed help explaining to welfare that she could not work because of her illness, and later she became part of a group of Somali women getting skills training, which helped with her socialization a great deal. Throughout that time, she was treated primarily with antidepressants and changing regimens of antipsychotics. Aripiprazole appears to have helped the best, and she is taking that currently.

This case is interesting because the patient has had multiple traumas, but they were never the focus of the treatment, partly because her overwhelming reactions to her children's problems and behaviors, and later her own psychosis, needed much more clinical attention.

Unlike IPT, our approach is not time limited but open-ended, because experience has indicated that most patients have symptoms that fluctuate with stress. Our sessions are scheduled for a half hour, usually every few weeks after initial evaluation but less frequently as patients settle in. The counselors have a good understanding of each of their patients and bring them in more frequently during crisis.

The following case illustrates how existing trauma reactivates and adds to previous trauma.

Case 2

The patient is a 60-year-old Bosnian man who has been in the United States 20 years. He reports having very poor sleep and experiencing nightmares three or four times per night. His current symptoms started about 18 months ago when an industrial accident crushed his pelvis, and since that time he has not been able to work and is in constant pain. The nightmares involve the current trauma as well as traumas related to the Bosnian situation. He only gets 3–4 hours of sleep per night and is very irritable. The patient experienced multiple traumas in Bosnia. The town he lived in was burned down, and the men were separated from the women by Serbian soldiers. Sixty-five men were killed on the spot. The women and the children were forced away, and for 14 months he did not know where his family was. He later escaped by going to a town that was unfortunately the focus of severe genocide. He was able to escape from that town, but he could not explain exactly what happened. The traumas included enduring physical beatings, witnessing murders, going without food, and observing the genocide in at least two places. He obviously has pain and walks with a cane, but he tells his story in a straightforward way. He admits he gets reactivated as he describes his trauma history. He does seem to get depressed at times and slightly agitated; there is no evidence of delusions or hallucinations.

This man has been followed up in therapy now for almost 2 years. He is seen every 4–6 weeks. Primary issues that are dealt with in psychotherapy are the complicated issues of dealing with workers' compensation. After originally helping him, the workers' comp program deemed that he was not injured anymore and should probably go back to work, even with possibly pelvic fractures. This angered him a great deal. We dealt with workers' comp staff directly to try to help him, but we were not successful. Over time, this patient has become less irritable. Antidepressant medication and clonidine have helped his sleep improve, and the medication has also helped to diminish the nightmares, although he continues to experience them periodically, both from the Bosnian genocide and the industrial trauma.

The following case shows that with existing trauma there comes the reactivation of PTSD across often long intervals of remission.

Case 3

The patient is a Bosnian man, originally seen in our clinic 17 years ago, who at intake had only been in the United States 3 months. He complained of insomnia, nightmares of violence at least four times a week, intrusive thoughts about the war, startle reaction, irritability, poor memory, and poor concentration. During the war in Bosnia, he was held as a prisoner of war, was beaten himself, and saw others killed. Later, when he joined the Bosnian army, he suffered a shrapnel wound and was present at the massacre of Srebrenica. As a result of the wound, he required abdominal and bladder surgery.

The patient was treated for PTSD for 2 years, then dropped out of treatment, and the last notes indicated he was doing quite well. This patient returned 3 years later complaining of many of the same symptoms. He had not been taking medicine since he left the clinic, and all the symptoms he previously experienced had returned. There was no new stress that he was aware of. He stayed in treatment for about 7 years and then dropped out again.

Seven years later he returned with the same symptoms. He had been doing well until about a year before the current visit, when the symptoms started again. These included nightmares, which occurred frequently if he saw violence on television or if he talked about the Bosnian situation with his friends. At these times, he would get very poor sleep, and he would notice a little agitation, which he can control now. Sometimes he felt sad and hopeless, but he was not suicidal. As with the last time, he was started on imipramine and clonidine, and at follow-up after several months he was doing quite well.

It is clear the patient had two expressions of symptoms recurring several years apart, with improvement each time, and no acute stress accounting for symptom recurrence. He is now committed to taking at least some medicine for a much longer period, because the exacerbations of symptoms have been quite difficult for him.

Postmigration factors can add to the original symptoms and can reactivate symptoms after a period of remission. These periods of stress become the primary issues of therapy.

THERAPIST FACTORS IN THERAPY

Many techniques or approaches to treatment of PTSD seem to minimize the role of therapist. Research on the therapist variable in therapy outcomes shows that factors such as warmth, genuineness, and trustworthiness account for more variance than the technique (Dalenberg 2014). IPT research demonstrates that the quality of the therapeutic relationship (i.e., friendliness) predicts better outcomes in that approach (Zuroff et al. 2017).

Our program's psychiatrists and ethnic counselors uniformly have empathetic and genuine concerns for refugees, and the relationship with their patients is characterized by friendliness and gentle humor. Undoubtedly, this relationship is the single most important factor in successful therapy with refugees.

I have described specific issues in psychotherapy of traumatized refugees in another report (Kinzie 2001), but I will augment that report with the following suggestions, indicating special qualities needed in therapists who are working with refugees.

Patients have a need to tell their story, and the psychiatrist has a need to listen, despite how painful it is for both parties. This process requires much uninterrupted time with a nonjudgmental approach. On many occasions, patients have never revealed their pain and shame before. To be accepted and believed in a nonjudgmental way provides powerful relief and cements the relationship. The ability of psychiatrists to listen is a necessary part of the healing process. It is also very difficult for some psychiatrists to do.

Case 4

The patient is a middle-aged, well-educated African woman. She described the trauma she experienced when gangs came to her town and began killing men, including her husband. She slowly improved with treatment, and after several months of treatment she asked the counselor to leave the room. Then she spoke to me in fair English. She said that what she had described was not all—she had been gang raped. She said that she felt dirty and was unable to talk about it to anyone. I said little and gave her a hug. We never talked about it again, but she seemed relieved and more open in subsequent interviews.

CONSISTENCY

Patients who are refugees need consistency and predictability over time. The constant and predictable relationship established by the psychiatrist is a reassuring factor. Refugees have faced much uncertainty—during war; in refugee camps; and in interactions with immigration officials, welfare workers, and neighbors—and having their doctor and counselor always be there in a place of safety and acceptance as essential. Many patients stay in treatment for a long time because it is the only place where they can be unafraid and a totally accepted person in American society. The psychiatrist is required to always be on time, consistent, and reliable in approach, and to remember with each patient the basic stresses the patient has faced and the previous interactions.

THE PROBLEM OF EVIL

Many patients have faced the most extreme traumas known (forced labor, starvation, and death of family and friends during the Pol Pot regime; long wars in Somalia, with indiscriminate killings, starvation, and even further abuse, robbery, and rape in refugee camps; mass murder in Bosnia, to name a few examples). These are not just crimes against individuals; they are crimes against humanity and are evil deeds. Patients explicitly, and sometimes implicitly, ask how people can do these things to other people. The question about evil is often raised and deserves a response, but it is unclear what the response should be. Agreeing that an evil occurred and that no one should have to be subjected to it seems to be a minimal response. Beyond that, responses fail. Perhaps it is genuine to state, "It is evil. I'm sorry that it happened to you, and I don't know why." It is an incomplete but honest answer and hopefully one that helps patients and psychiatrists alike.

COUNTERTRANSFERENCE ISSUES

Countertransference (another term for the condition is "empathetic strain" or perhaps more accurately "empathetic overload") occurs often in psychotherapy with traumatized patients. After one hears stories of human violence toward other humans, it is impossible not to feel both irritable and overwhelmed by the sheer magnitude of the manifest evil in the world. I have evaluated and treated more than 1,200 refugees and asylum seekers over 40 years. However, having too many intakes in a row (i.e., more than two a week) sometimes proves a tipping point for me, coupled with feelings of frustration, irritability, and vicarious nightmares. Our counselors—many of whom have had traumatic personal experiences—have an added stress as they reexperience their own traumas while translating the patients' stories. These feelings of frustration and stress pass in time as patients settle in and start expressing relief and gratitude. What makes it possible to continue is that patients get better.

Their sleep improves, their nightmares decrease, and their irritability is reduced; they proceed with daily activities, and they are making a living and raising a family. The difficulties and symptoms are not over, and they will probably get worse at times. However, they have confidence that we will continue to be there for them. Their gratitude and appreciation are genuine—a smile, a handshake, and a wish to me that I myself will have a good day. This is one of the rewards of working with refugees.

Psychiatrists need to do this valuable work, but they must also prevent burn out. Not all psychiatrists and counselors feel this kind of reward. Multiple requests for letters, information about medicine, lab tests, and even discussions about how to take the bus system can be tedious and frustrating. This tedium can, and sometimes does, lead to a high burnout rate among treatment providers working with torture survivors. For most psychiatrists, providing treatment to a very seriously ill patient population is part of the demanding job that we have chosen and for which we have been trained. Our professional dedication keeps us involved, and patients' improvement provides our rewards.

Case 5

The patient is a gentle, highly respected Bosnian man of 50 who had spent several years in a Serbian concentration camp. He reported seeing many atrocities, including murder and starvation. He reported witnessing a guard give a man a piece of bread, who rapidly ate it and ignored his starving son. The patient was appalled by the father's selfish cruelty. The patient only survived when a guard recognized him and took him out alone and let him escape. After his escape, he met his in-laws and asked them to leave to another country. They refused and were killed the next day.

He had been a patient for a year when he decided to tell us that what he had described was not all he had seen. He and other prisoners were forced to clean out bodies of murdered Bosnians from their homes, to make room for Serbs. In the pile of bodies in one home a little blonde girl appeared hands up and crying. The patient picked up the little girl, took her to a guard, and asked, "What should we do?" The guard grabbed the little girl and threw her against a tree and killed her. After telling the story, the patient bowed his head and said nothing. The Bosnian counselor appeared stunned and wiped away a tear. I think I thanked him for telling the difficult experience. However, our feelings were a mixture of sorrow for the patient, who carried the burden of this tragedy; anger at the murderous guard and all Serbs who indiscriminately killed many Bosnians; but mostly grief about a little girl sitting in a group of bodies, probably including those of her own parents, and asking for help, then being killed. A life cut short. The evil without justice leaves one with a sense of helplessness. Overall, after the anger is sadness about our patient and the little unknown girl, and a war that encouraged murders of "the enemies." After talking for a little more time and conveying my care nonverbally, the counselor and I respectfully acknowledged his pain, and we continued the session. But I could not forget the trauma the patient had experienced, and I remained depressed and irritable for some time.

CURRENT POLITICAL ATMOSPHERE

At the time of writing this chapter, there is a general unease, if not pessimism, overlaying all refugee treatment. The rejection of asylum seekers, the rapid deportation of many immigrants, the refusal to allow Muslim refugees into the country, and the separation of children from parents at borders, speak to an official hostility toward refugees and asylum seekers. This hostility is not just for refugees and asylum seekers; it also affects legal immigrants in efforts to get citizenship. There are now even plans to review those who have already obtained U.S. citizenship, making these persons feel that their position as a U.S. citizen is vulnerable. Hate groups have more license to hate or attack refugees, particularly those of color. There is no denying that tolerance of diversity is waning, and refugees are somewhat in the line of fire. This is a reality and represents a limit on what we can do to help people. The pressure is always there, and it is sometimes expressed openly by patients. How to respond to their concerns is not clear either. Perhaps agreeing with them that they are under continued observation and perhaps subject to more overt prejudice than previously is a confirming aspect to their own experience. Outside the therapy session, taking more direct political action is an option for many people. The current political climate can make these tasks seem overwhelming.

Case 6

This patient is an African American patient who is not a refugee. She is well educated and intelligent and has felt very comfortable in her role in the community until the last 2 years. She has seen more demonstrated prejudice against African Americans and refugees and has felt more personal danger. She has even thought about carrying a gun at times. Over the past few years, the change in her behavior has been obvious, and she is no longer as high-spirited and easygoing. She comments to me, "If *I* feel the threat, how much more must refugees feel it?"

CONCLUSION

Psychotherapy is an important part of the total treatment of traumatized refugees. It needs to be combined with pharmacotherapy, social therapy, and aid in such causes as helping with asylum and citizenship, ensuring good medical care, assisting with finding employment, helping pursue language education, and obtaining medical disability benefits, when indicated. These individuals face multiple issues of stress and losses, resulting in several common psychiatric diagnoses, namely PTSD and depression. Also, there is the need for consistent language interpretation and cultural understanding to make a meaningful therapeutic contact. There is no universal approach to fit all refugees, but in our experience, helping patients deal with postmigration stresses, rather than providing trauma (usually traumas)–focused therapy, is the priority. The most important issue is for the psychiatrist and the mental health counselor to develop a long-term relationship with the refugee patient based on respect and empathy.

KEY CLINICAL POINTS

- Although many, if not most, refugee patients have experienced severe trauma, initial trauma-focused therapy may miss the ongoing postmigration problems of adjusting to a new culture.
- Ongoing stresses may reactivate the prior trauma and are the focus of long-term therapy.
- The focus of therapy is to deal with everyday stresses of language, poverty, children's conflicts, and, sometimes, discrimination.
- The clinic with psychiatrists and counselors from the patient's culture may be the most stable part of his or her life because it provides ongoing consistency in an unsettled time of the refugee's life.
- The psychiatrist's characteristics of consistency, empathy, and warmth are the most important aspects of treatment.
- Confronting the problem of evil (e.g., hearing stories of the utter cruelty of human beings to other human beings) may stretch the empathy of the psychiatrist, but helping the patient get well provides hope to continue this important work.

REFERENCES

Bruhn M, Rees S, Mohsin M, et al: The range and impact of postmigration stressors during treatment of trauma-affected refugees. J Nerv Ment Dis 206(1):61–68, 2018 29194088

Charney ME, Hellberg SN, Bui E, et al: Evidenced-based treatment of posttraumatic stress disorder: an updated review of validated psychotherapeutic and pharmacological approaches. Harv Rev Psychiatry 26(3):99–115, 2018 29734225

Dalenberg CJ: On building a science of common factors in trauma therapy. J Trauma Dissociation 15(4):373–383, 2014 24979256

Kinzie JD: Psychotherapy for massively traumatized refugees: the therapist variable. Am J Psychother 55(4):475–490, 2001 11824215

Markowitz JC, Petkova E, Neria Y, et al: Is exposure necessary? A randomized clinical trial of interpersonal psychotherapy for PTSD. Am J Psychiatry 172(5):430–440, 2015 25677355

Nickerson A, Bryant RA, Silove D, et al: A critical review of psychological treatment of posttraumatic stress disorder in refugees. Clin Psychol Rev 31(3):399–417, 2011 25677355

Nickerson A, Schick M, Schnyder U, et al: Comorbidity of posttraumatic stress disorder and depression in tortured, treatment-seeking refugees. J Trauma Stress 30(4):409–415, 2017 21112681

Schoch K, Böttche M, Rosner R, et al: Impact of new traumatic or stressful life events on pre-existing PTSD in traumatized refugees: results of a longitudinal study. Eur J Psychotraumatol 7:32106, 2016 27834172

Thompson CT, Vidgen A, Roberts NP: Psychological interventions for posttraumatic stress disorder in refugees and asylum seekers: a systematic review and meta-analysis. Clin Psychol Rev 63:66–79, 2018 29936342

Zuroff DC, McBride C, Ravitz P, et al: Autonomous and controlled motivation for interpersonal therapy for depression: between-therapists and within-therapist effects. J Couns Psychol 64(5):525–537, 2017 29048189

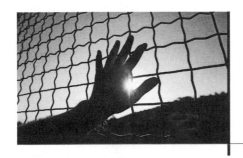

Chapter 5

PSYCHOBIOLOGY AND PSYCHOPHARMACOLOGY

J. David Kinzie, M.D., FACPsych, DLFAPA

The most common diagnosis of a refugee patient in a psychiatry clinic is PTSD, with rates approaching 100% among Cambodians. This is not surprising because most refugees have endured periods of civil war, witnessed genocide, experienced starvation and torture, and lived through deaths of family members by violence. In addition, most have been in unsafe refugee camps prior to coming to the United States, some for as long as 15 years. In refugees, PTSD is a comorbid condition with depression, with this comorbidity occurring in, on average, about 80% in this population. For example, a chart review of 50 African patients found that among 34 patients with PTSD, 31 also had depression (91% comorbidity rate) (Cannon 1932). The comorbid depression is undoubtedly related to refugee losses—related to family, country, social standing, and occupational position—as well as to humiliation from police and gangs while in refugee camps. Loss, humiliation, and entrapment have been found to be related to depression (Brown et al. 1995). Additionally,

59

about 10% of our clinic patients have psychosis, usually including schizophrenia. Some of the psychotic symptoms started after exposure to multiple traumas.

PSYCHOBIOLOGY

Since Cannon's 1932 description of the fight-or-flight reaction to threat, it is well recognized that the body reacts to threat and danger. Since 1980, when the criteria for PTSD were first included in DSM (in DSM-III; American Psychiatric Association 1980), much research has gone into defining the CNS changes that occur in reaction to trauma. The findings are somewhat confusing and contradictory, but I will summarize the most consistent findings that are clinically relevant. Excellent reviews of these findings have been provided by Pitman et al. (2012) and Sherin and Nemeroff (2011) and are recommended for additional readings.

Functional imaging has demonstrated several important CNS changes in patients with PTSD. The amygdala, which plays a role in fear reactions, shows increased activity under threatening stimuli. The ventral medial prefrontal cortex shows decreased activation to trauma-related stimuli. The dorsal anterior cingulate cortex, involved in fear learning, shows increased activity in PTSD patients with fear conditioning.

NORADRENERGIC STUDIES

Despite the many advances in understanding the neurobiology of PTSD, little of these have resulted in rational drug treatment. The exception is a noradrenergic dysregulation in PTSD. High levels of noradrenergic activity are related to hyperarousal, nightmares, and poor sleep (De Berardis et al. 2015; Hendrickson and Raskind 2016). Furthermore, noradrenergic receptor blockers and receptor antagonists, which reduce norepinephrine in the locus coeruleus and amygdala, can reduce hyperarousal symptoms and nightmares. The α_2-adrenergic receptors are spread throughout the CNS but specifically are found in the pontine locus coeruleus (Naguy 2016). α_2-Agonist agents have sedation analgesia and vasodilatation effects but little effect on the respiratory drive and therefore have a good safety record. Clinically clonidine is an older drug used to treat hypertension, ADHD (Joo and Kim 2018), and opioid use disorder (Toce et al. 2018). Clonidine has also been used in the treatment of nightmares and hyperarousal associated with PTSD, and we have used it for over 30 years (Boehnlein and Kinzie 2007). Prazosin and another adrenergic antagonist, doxazosin (an α_1 receptor antagonist), have been effective in the treatment of nightmares and hyper-arousal symptoms (Roepke et al. 2017). Although a recent report has questioned the effectiveness of prazosin based on results from a randomized trial (Raskind et al. 2018), much clinical experience indicates it is effective.

SYMPATHETIC CNS STUDIES

Norepinephrine

There is strong evidence for sympathetic nervous system hyperactivity in PTSD, including increased blood levels of norepinephrine and the development of hypertension. A PET study evaluating the availability of norepinephrine in the locus coeruleus found that norepinephrine transporter availability was positively correlated with PTSD hyperarousal symptoms (Pietrzak et al. 2013).

Serotonin

The role of serotonin (5-HT) is complicated, but one factor in the vulnerability to PTSD is a variation of a gene that codes for *serotonin transporter*, also known as a *serotonin uptake site*. A study on Rwandan genocide survivors found that those with the short form (SS) of the promotor serotonin transporter gene would develop PTSD after very few traumatic events (Kolassa et al. 2010). A review of the literature on the short form of the serotonin transporter gene found that this polymorphism represents a risk factor of PTSD in patients with high trauma exposure (Gressier et al. 2013). The emerging evidence seems to point to a risk effect of the serotonin transporter gene coupled with trauma (i.e., adversity), which can result in PTSD (McGuffin et al. 2011).

Cortisol

Unlike in acute stress, in which cortisol levels are elevated, in PTSD cortisol levels are either low or normal. This surprising effect is thought to be due to the negative feedback sensitivity of the hypothalamic-pituitary-adrenal axis (Pitman et al. 2012).

NEUROCIRCUITRY

Multiple lines of evidence from PTSD studies implicate bilateral amygdala and anterior cingulate cortex hyperactivity and ventral medial prefrontal cortex (VMPFC) hypoactivity in PTSD. There is a reciprocal relationship between the amygdala and VMPFC; during times of stress, the amygdala becomes hyperactive and is not inhibited by the VMPFC. The amygdala also activates the locus coeruleus, and this results in increased sympathetic activity. A review of imaging studies involving PTSD patients who responded to therapy showed that functional changes result in decreased amygdala and increased dorsal prefrontal activation (Thomaes et al. 2014).

PHARMACOLOGICAL TREATMENT OF TRAUMATIZED REFUGEES

ROLE OF MEDICATION

After the original interview, which can be lengthy because the history may involve multiple traumas, a diagnosis can be listed. The next step, rather than going on to treatment planning, is to ask, "What are the symptoms you most want to be relieved from?" In my clinical experience, the most important symptoms our refugee patients have are poor sleep (for many years), persistent nightmares, and agitation, which can be disruptive to the family. A simple explanation of the course of the symptoms, an example of which is presented below, can be helpful for patients to understand the disorder and relieve a sense of "going crazy":

> You had a very difficult life with some severe, bad experiences [I then mention some of them]. And even though you are strong, your body wears down, and now you have poor sleep, nightmares, and flashbacks and you are irritated. This is understandable, and we can help you feel better.

It is necessary to explain to patients what medicine can and cannot do. It cannot bring back family members who have died, it cannot restore the community and culture, and it cannot even provide an understanding of why the evil occurred. It can, however, help with sleep and reduce nightmares, hyperarousal, depression, and irritability. At the end, I ask if the patient has any questions. There usually are a few questions, but sometimes I'm asked whether the medicine is addicting, and I clarify that the medicine we use is not. In a typical case of PTSD and depression, we start the patient on medicine and explain that the purpose is to help improve the mood and sleep and reduce flashbacks. The patient is told that people differ and that some will need more and some less medicine and that the amount will be adjusted as needed. I also tell them to call the counselor with any problems and we can talk and I will advise what to do. Obviously, the therapeutic relationship is a basic part of treatment itself, but a strong alliance also helps to ensure compliance.

COMPLIANCE

Compliance varies with patients' cultures. When we started our clinic almost 40 years ago, we studied blood levels of an antidepressant and found that very few patients had adequate serum levels of medicine. In fact, some ethnic groups, such as the Cambodians, had no detectable level of the antidepressant (Kinzie and Leung 1989). With education and encouragement from the counselors, compliance increased, as did the treatment response. Offering group sessions where medicine is discussed by patients themselves effectively conveys information and modeling for the new patients. Many patients, despite being advised not to, will stop their medicine when their prescriptions run out. It sometimes takes several sessions to educate patients on the importance of maintenance treatment and the need to get prescriptions refilled. Although there are exceptions, refugee patients from ethnic groups require doses similar to those American patients receive in order to have a therapeutic response.

LENGTH OF TREATMENT

Severely traumatized refugees with depression and PTSD have a chronic course with exacerbation and remissions, and require long-term treatment. Therefore, we counsel patients on their treatment with paradoxical advice: "You will get better, and you need to stay in treatment." Commonly, patients whose condition is reasonably stable will relapse, usually with PTSD symptoms. The precipitant is almost always a new trigger stimulus—hearing news of death or fighting in their homeland, watching news or violence on television (the 9/11 event is a prime example), witnessing an accident where blood is evident, experiencing the death of a friend or acquaintance—all bring back the original traumas. An explanation of the triggering process is helpful, as is a temporary increase of medicine. Many patients consider themselves vulnerable and continue with psychotherapy and medicine to preserve stability and prevent relapse. Not uncommonly, many patients who drop out of treatment return with a new onset of symptoms. We have had people in continuous treatment for over 25 years.

CULTURAL ISSUES IN DRUG TREATMENT

Special Considerations

Despite being from different cultures (our clinic treats patients from 18 different language groups), traumatized patients seem much more similar than different. A few generalizations are in order. Ramadan, a Muslim religious time lasting about 1 month with no food or water intake allowed during daylight hours, requires that medicines prescribed during daytime not be taken. For these patients, as much as possible, medications should be prescribed to be taken in the evening before bedtime. Appointment times must be flexible. Africans tend not to adhere to the regular appointment time, although they usually come in the same day. Bosnians follow European tradition and are usually right on time and rarely fail to show up at appointments. Many patients from rural areas in Asia and Africa are illiterate and cannot read the labels of medicine and need repeated explanations and reminders to take medicine. A pill box is very helpful, especially if multiple medicines for other disorders, such as diabetes and hypertension, are prescribed.

Drug treatment in refugees is predicated on a therapeutic relationship, an understanding of the patient's culture with help from a culturally appropriate interpreter, to establish a diagnosis and negotiate a treatment plan. The plan should improve target goals and information about medicines. It should not be short-term, it needs to include psychotherapy with a psychiatrist, and it should be hopeful yet realistic. As one patient put it, "I am much better, but I still have some nightmares, and I will for the rest of my life." Massive trauma for refugees is enduring.

There are cultural problems associated with treating refugees with psychiatric medications. Many patients from Asia believe that American medicine is too strong and cut the dose in half. Most have no understanding of the long-term use of medicines and stop taking them as soon as the prescription is finished or as soon as they feel better. Education about medicine, often in a group setting, is helpful. Of course, medicine is only part of the treatment program, which includes social interventions and psychotherapy. With that in mind, medicine can usually bring rapidly improve sleep and much reduced nightmares and irritability, helping the very troubled patients.

Drug Abuse and Alcohol Use Disorder

Refugees in our clinic are mostly Buddhist or Muslim and have low rates of drug abuse or suicide. We have a few patients with drug and alcohol problems, primarily the children of first-generation immigrants. Suicide is also very rare. In 40 years of treatment, we have had five deaths from suicide, all involving patients with schizophrenia. Despite suffering severe traumas as adults, very few patients have personality disorders. The absence of substance use disorders and suicidal threats makes treatments with medications easier and safer.

SPECIFIC MEDICATION SUGGESTIONS

Our own group has used noradrenergic-blocking agents for over 30 years and has found them to be effective in reducing nightmares and other hyperarousal symptoms (Boehnlein and Kinzie 2007). The dose range of prazosin is 2 to 10 mg usually given at bedtime. Clonidine is effective in promoting sleep because of its sedative properties, and it additionally reduces nightmares and hyperarousal symptoms (Boehnlein and Kinzie 2007; Kinzie and Leung 1989; Morgenthaler et al. 2018). The dose range for clonidine is 0.2 to 0.9 mg given at bedtime.

Although not usual, the following case examples illustrate that these agents can be effective as monotherapy for PTSD.

Case 1

A 25-year-old woman from a Mayan-speaking indigenous group in Central America suffered significant trauma during the Guatemalan Civil War. She witnessed guerillas kill her father, her mother was raped and burned to death, four brothers were killed, and she was thrown to the ground and thought to be dead. She fled to Mexico but was raped by a family friend and suffered flashbacks of both that assault and previous traumas. When seen at the clinic, she was found to have severe PTSD with nightmares every night. She was started on prazosin, but because of side effects a switch was made to clonidine. Within 7 months, her symptoms were reduced and her nightmares were gone. During follow-up for the next 7 years, she continued taking only clonidine. She was asymptomatic without nightmares, and the irritability and startle reaction stopped. Relationships with her family greatly improved. She is maintained on 0.1 mg clonidine currently.

Case 2

A 37-year-old Cambodian man, first seen at the clinic in 1994, had experienced massive trauma in Cambodia, including his father being executed by the Pol Pot regime, his mother dying of illness during the Pol Pot regime, people being taken for execution, and he himself being taken and beaten into unconsciousness. He had many problems with nightmares two to three times per week and many symptoms of depression with insomnia.

During the next 2 years, he was started on various antidepressants and on clonidine. Seven years later, the nightmares were better but continued. He then was started on prazosin with citalopram, and clonidine was discontinued. Prazosin was increased, and 9 years later he was taking prazosin 10 mg at night. Later, all medications except prazosin were stopped, and for the last 10 years he has been taking only prazosin. He has been completely free of nightmares for the last 15 years while taking only 5 mg of prazosin.

SSRI and SNRI Antidepressants

The selective serotonin reuptake inhibitors (SSRIs) paroxetine and sertraline are the only FDA-approved drugs for PTSD. Fluoxetine and the serotonin-norepinephrine reuptake inhibitor venlafaxine may also help major PTSD symptoms. The effect sizes in studies of these first-line medicines tend to be small (Hoskins et al. 2015). Less than 30% of studied patients attained full remission (Kelmendi et al. 2016). A systematic study of treatment for refugees concluded that no specific pharmacological treatment could be recommended (Sonne et al. 2017). On the other hand, a study of Bosnian refugees found that sertraline and paroxetine were effective in both PTSD and depression symptoms (Smajkić et al. 2001).

Tricyclic Antidepressants

From 1950 through 1980 tricyclic antidepressants (TCAs) were the primary antidepressants available to psychiatrists. However, with newer medicines such as SSRIs, the TCAs have fallen out of favor (Chockalingam et al. 2019). It is now argued that TCAs should play a role especially in treatment-resistant depression (Navarro et al. 2019) and melancholic depression (Valerio et al. 2018). In the Rapp model treatment, with imipramine and fluoxetine, fluoxetine reverses the depressive-like phenotype, whereas imipramine reestablishes hippocampal neurogenesis and neuronal dendrite arborization. These effects may contribute to the resilience of TCAs in recurrent depression (Alves et al. 2017).

The TCAs, such as imipramine, are classified, in neuroscience-base nomenclature, as a serotonin-norepinephrine reuptake inhibitor. They are FDA-approved for depression but also prescribed for anxiety, insomnia, and chronic pain (Stahl 2017). Their action is related to blocking the serotonin and norepinephrine pump and increasing serotonin and adrenergic transmission. Imipramine also blocks α_1-adrenergic receptors, as do amitriptyline and doxepin, and this explains its sedative and hypotensive effects and also the reduction in nightmares and hyperarousal. Davidson (2015) has argued that TCAs have advantages in PTSD, including in the treatment of comorbid depression, insomnia, and pain.

One of the most common complaints among our PTSD patients is problems with sleep, with some patients getting only a few hours at night, lasting for several years. Recurrent nightmares cause frequent awakening with severe anxiety. TCAs such as imipramine and doxepin, when combined with clonidine or prazosin, are used to treat depression, insomnia, and nightmares. A caution in this combination includes the fact that TCAs may reduce the hypotensive effect of clonidine, although clonidine is not being used solely as a hypertensive agent in our experience. TCAs can be fatal in severe overdoses. We have had not had any overdoses in 40 years of experience with TCAs. This probably is because Muslims and Buddhists, our largest patient groups, have religious prohibitions against suicide. TCAs are not used in older patients because of the risk of dementia (Wang et al. 2018). The maintenance dose of imipramine and of doxepin is 100–150 mg taken at night. I have advocated for the combination of TCAs and clonidine for treatment of traumatized refugees (Kinzie 2016).

Case 3

A 38-year-old Cambodian woman was struggling with anger, frequent nightmares (almost nightly), depression, and reexperiencing of the death of her siblings. During the Pol Pot regime, she was separated from her family; her brother was executed, her mother died of starvation, and the patient was threatened with death and saw many others killed and starved. Only the Vietnamese invasion saved her life. She was diagnosed with severe PTSD and major depression and was started on imipramine 50 mg and clonidine 0.4 mg at bedtime. The imipramine was increased to 150 mg and later changed to doxepin. She has continued to take doxepin and clonidine for 25 years. She continues to do well, coming three to four times per year for clinic appointments and socialization activities. She is very stable now, has no nightmares, and, by her own choice, continues taking the same medication regimen.

Case 4

A 37-year-old man was first seen in 2001 when he was a new immigrant to the United States. In Bosnia, he experienced the war and was held in a detention center and beaten. He saw others beaten and killed, and he was injured severely when a bomb exploded; he had to have surgery to remove shrapnel from his abdomen and bladder. He described hiding out in the woods while 34 other men in his village, including his father and brother, were killed. He had irritability, nightmares, and startle reaction. He was treated for PTSD and major depression. He felt better and dropped out of treatment after 2 years. He returned 3 years later with nightmares, intrusive thoughts, and irritability. He was in treatment for 5 more years after resumption of PTSD symptoms, then dropped out for 5 years. In 2018, he returned with no precipitating reason; he developed more nightmares, two to three times per night, and had very poor sleep, only 4–5 hours a night, and a little irritability. He was restarted on the same medication as before: imipramine 100 mg and clonidine 0.4 mg, both at bedtime. Within a month his sleep improved and the nightmares decreased greatly, and he continues in treatment at this time.

Atypical Antipsychotics

Irritability and aggression are the third most common complaints after poor sleep and nightmares. We have used risperidone in our clinic, and literature also suggests it is helpful with irritability. More recently, aripiprazole has been advocated as monotherapy. A review of the literature found that PTSD symptoms have a good response to aripiprazole (Britnell et al. 2017). We have used aripiprazole both for aggressive behavior or irritability and for augmentation of antidepressant response (see Case Study 5).

About 10% of our patients have psychotic symptoms or schizophrenia. Because of the high occurrence of diabetes in refugee groups, we have attempted to stay away from the second generation of antipsychotics and often use first-generation medications, such as perphenazine.

Case 5

The patient is a Bosnian woman, who during the war in Bosnia, experienced many terrible events. She saw seven people killed and went without food for a long time. Her father was killed by a bomb, although she did not see it. She saw soldiers killing children. Because of her unusual thought processes, it was very difficult to get a history of her trauma. Her speech was rather odd and somewhat tangential. It was clear she had PTSD and depression, but at a follow-up appointment 1 month later she had more anger, hallucinations of hearing her mother calling her name, and yelling that was disrupting her family. Her speech was rapidly changing and disorganized. She was started on risperidone, which was later changed to perphenazine and imipramine. For the past 12 years, she has been taking imipramine 100 mg and perphenazine 32 mg both at bedtime. She has been quite stable on that regimen. The psychotic symptoms are gone, and she rarely has any other symptoms, including nightmares.

About 10% of our patients have psychotic symptoms, and about half of these are diagnosed with schizophrenia. We have found that intramuscular long-acting medicine has been useful in attaining compliance for many patients. Surprisingly, the patients come quite regularly to get their injections and do very well. We have had very few hospitalizations of patients on intramuscular medicine. We originally used fluphenazine decanoate, with most patients doing very well. Currently, many patients have been started on paliperidone (Invega), which is a little less flexible to use but seems to have fewer side effects. Currently we have about 50 patients who are receiving intramuscular medicine regularly.

FUTURE DIRECTIONS

It is now known that inflammation plays a role in depression and PTSD. Biomedical markers of inflammation, such as elevated C-reactive protein (CRP) and WBC, which are easily measured, have been shown to predict a poorer course of PTSD and depression (Eswarappa et al. 2019).

There is some evidence that CRP level may predict antidepressant response (Hughes and Kumari 2017). A study found that augmenting the antidepressant with the anti-inflammatory medication celecoxib can increase the antidepressant response (Edberg et al. 2018).

It may be useful, or even necessary, soon to have inflammatory markers, such as WBC or CRP, to aid in the treatment of PTSD and depression.

CONCLUSION

The cases in this chapter illustrate that treatment of tortured refugees is long-term and that many patients suffer remissions and exacerbations. However, pharmacotherapy is quite successful in symptom reduction.

Many refugees suffer trauma in their countries of origin and in refugee camps and develop PTSD, major depression, and sometimes psychosis. Pharmacological therapy can treat their symptoms effectively, if given long-term. The adrenergic receptor–blocking agents prazosin, doxazosin, and clonidine can alleviate the nightmares and hyperarousal symptoms. Although SSRIs are recommended for PTSD, in our population we found that TCAs, particularly imipramine and doxepin, help with depression and sleep. Agitation can be relieved by risperidone and aripiprazole. In many refugee clinics, effective pharmacotherapy is underutilized, and I recommend that more extensive and appropriate use of medications could help many symptoms of these troubled patients.

KEY CLINICAL POINTS

- Traumatized refugees with PTSD and depression have many symptoms and complaints that can be helped by medicine.

- Within the context of a therapeutic relationship and with a clear explanation of the purpose of the medicine, refugee patients can accept and are compliant with medicine.

- The two most common complaints from refugees are poor sleep and very frequent nightmares, occurring with depression. Clonidine and prazosin are effective in reducing nightmares. Although the selective serotonin reuptake inhibitors sertraline and paroxetine are approved for PTSD, the sedative tricyclics imipramine and doxepin are effective with clonidine or prazosin for improving sleep and reducing nightmares.

- Agitation and irritability are important symptoms and can be treated with risperidone and aripiprazole.
- Psychosis and sometimes frank schizophrenia should be treated with regular antipsychotic medicine. Caution needs to be exercised with second-generation antipsychotics because the prevalence of diabetes is already high in this population.
- Treatment needs to be long term, because PTSD among refugees is a chronic, relapsing disorder.

REFERENCES

Alves ND, Correia JS, Patrício P, et al: Adult hippocampal neuroplasticity triggers susceptibility to recurrent depression. Transl Psychiatry Mar 14;7(3):e1058, 2017 28291258

American Psychiatric Association: Diagnostic and Statistical Manual of Mental Disorders, 3rd Edition. Washington, DC, American Psychiatric Association, 1980

Boehnlein JK, Kinzie JD: Pharmacologic reduction of CNS noradrenergic activity in PTSD: the case for clonidine and prazosin. J Psychiatr Pract 13(2):72–78, 2007 17414682

Britnell SR, Jackson AD, Brown JN, et al: Aripiprazole for post-traumatic stress disorder: a systematic review. Clin Neuropharmacol 40(6):273–278, 2017 29059134

Brown GW, Harris TO, Hepworth C: Loss, humiliation and entrapment among women developing depression: a patient and non-patient comparison. Psychol Med 25(1):7–21, 1995 7792364

Cannon WB: The Wisdom of the Body. New York, WW Norton, 1932

Chockalingam R, Gott BM, Conway CR: Tricyclic antidepressants and monoamine oxidase inhibitors: are they too old for a new look? Handb Exp Pharmacol 250:37–48, 2019 30105472

Davidson J: Vintage treatments for PTSD: a reconsideration of tricyclic drugs. J Psychopharmacol 29(3):264–269, 2015 25586404

De Berardis D, Marini S, Serroni N, et al: Targeting the noradrenergic system in posttraumatic stress disorder: a systematic review and meta-analysis of Prazosin trials. Curr Drug Targets 16(10):1094–1106, 2015 25944011

Edberg D, Hoppensteadt D, Walborn A, et al: Plasma C-reactive protein levels in bipolar depression during cyclooxygenase-2 inhibitor combination treatment. J Psychiatr Res 102:1–7, 2018 29554535

Eswarappa M, Neylan TC, Whooley MA, et al: Inflammation as a predictor of disease course in posttraumatic stress disorder and depression: a prospective analysis from the Mind Your Heart Study. Brain Behav Immun 75:220–227, 2019 30389462

Gressier F, Calati R, Balestri M, et al: The 5-HTTLPR polymorphism and posttraumatic stress disorder: a meta-analysis. J Trauma Stress 26(6):645–653, 2013 24222274

Hendrickson RC, Raskind MA: Noradrenergic dysregulation in the pathophysiology of PTSD. Exp Neurol 284(Pt B):181–195, 2016 27222130

Hoskins M, Pearce J, Bethell A, et al: Pharmacotherapy for post-traumatic stress disorder: systematic review and meta-analysis. Br J Psychiatry 206(2):93–100, 2015 25644881

Hughes A, Kumari M: Associations of C-reactive protein and psychological distress are modified by antidepressants, supporting an inflammatory depression subtype: findings from UKHLS. Brain Behav Immun 66:89–93, 2017 28728805

Joo SW, Kim HW: Treatment of children and adolescents with attention deficit hyperactivity disorder and/or Tourette's disorder with clonidine extended release. Psychiatry Investig 15(1):90–93, 2018 29422931

Kelmendi B, Adams TG, Yarnell S, et al: PTSD: from neurobiology to pharmacological treatments. Eur J Psychotraumatol 7:31858, 2016 27837583

Kinzie JD: Medical approach to management of traumatized refugees. J Psychiatr Pract 22(2):76–83, 2016 27138076

Kinzie JD, Leung P: Clonidine in Cambodian patients with posttraumatic stress disorder. J Nerv Ment Dis 177(9):546–550, 1989 2769247

Kolassa IT, Ertl V, Eckart C, et al: Association study of trauma load and SLC6A4 promoter polymorphism in posttraumatic stress disorder: evidence from survivors of the Rwandan genocide. J Clin Psychiatry 71(5):543–547, 2010 20441718

McGuffin P, Alsabban S, Uher R: The truth about genetic variation in the serotonin transporter gene and response to stress and medication. Br J Psychiatry 198(6):424–427, 2011 21628702

Morgenthaler TI, Auerbach S, Casey KR, et al: Position paper for the treatment of nightmare disorder in adults: an American Academy of Sleep Medicine position paper. J Clin Sleep Med 14(6):1041–1055, 2018 29852917

Naguy A: Clonidine use in psychiatry: panacea or panache. Pharmacology 98(1–2):87–92, 2016 27161101

Navarro V, Boulahfa I, Obach A, et al: Switching to imipramine versus add-on mirtazapine in venlafaxine-resistant major depression: a 10-week randomized open study. J Clin Psychopharmacol 39(1):63–66, 2019 30516574

Pietrzak RH, Gallezot JD, Ding YS, et al: Association of posttraumatic stress disorder with reduced in vivo norepinephrine transporter availability in the locus coeruleus. JAMA Psychiatry 70(11):1199–1205, 2013 24048210

Pitman RK, Rasmusson AM, Koenen KC, et al: Biological studies of posttraumatic stress disorder. Nat Rev Neurosci 13(11):769–787, 2012 23047775

Raskind MA, Peskind ER, Chow B, et al: Trial of prazosin for post-traumatic stress disorder in military veterans. N Engl J Med 308:510–517, 2018 29414272

Roepke S, Danker-Hopfe H, Repantis D, et al: Doxazosin, an α-1-adrenergic-receptor antagonist, for nightmares in patients with posttraumatic stress disorder and/or borderline personality disorder: a chart review. Pharmacopsychiatry 50(1):26–31, 2017 27276365

Sherin JE, Nemeroff CB: Post-traumatic stress disorder: the neurobiological impact of psychological trauma. Dialogues Clin Neurosci 13(3):263–278, 2011 22034143

Smajkić A, Weine S, Durić-Bijedić Z, et al: Sertraline, paroxetine and venlafaxine in refugee post traumatic stress disorder with depression symptoms. Med Arh 55(1)(Suppl 1):35–38, 2001 11795192

Sonne C, Carlsson J, Bech P, Mortensen EL: Pharmacological treatment of refugees with trauma-related disorders: what do we know today? Transcult Psychiatry 54(2):260–280, 2017 27956478

Stahl SM: Essential Psychopharmacology: Prescriber's Guide, 6th Edition. Cambridge, UK, Cambridge University Press, 2017, pp 341–347

Thomaes K, Dorrepaal E, Draijer N, et al: Can pharmacological and psychological treatment change brain structure and function in PTSD? A systematic review. J Psychiatr Res 50:1–15, 2014 24321592

Toce MS, Chai PR, Burns MM, et al: Pharmacologic treatment of opioid use disorder: a review of pharmacotherapy, adjuncts, and toxicity. J Med Toxicol 14(4):306–322, 2018 30377951

Valerio MP, Szmulewicz AG, Martino DJ: A quantitative review on outcome-to-antidepressants in melancholic unipolar depression. Psychiatry Res 265:100–110, 2018 29702301

Wang YC, Tai PA, Poly TN, et al: Increased risk of dementia in patients with antidepressants: a meta-analysis of observational studies. Behav Neurol Jul 10;2018:5315098, 2018 30123386

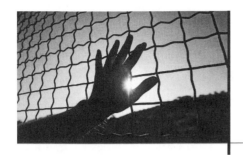

Chapter 6

THE OREGON MODEL

The Intercultural Psychiatric Program

J. David Kinzie, M.D., FACPsych, DLFAPA

In 1977, the department of psychiatry at Oregon Health & Science University (OHSU) established the Intercultural Psychiatric Program (IPP), a psychiatric program for refugees. The program is led by psychiatrists who are faculty members. However, the unique aspect of the Oregon model is its inclusion of full-time ethnic counselors and case managers, who serve as interpreters for the psychiatrist in treatment sessions with patients in their own ethnic group. This chapter adds to the original description of the program (Kinzie et al. 1980) and describes what we feel contributes to its longevity.

THE PATIENTS

Refugees are a diverse group, but they all have in common fleeing their own country and, usually, multiple traumatic experiences, including deaths of family members by violence, personal torture, periods of starvation, and prolonged time in unsafe refugee camps. Most do not know English and in the United States are easily overwhelmed by the confusing information about bureaucracy, housing, medical needs, education for children, and lack of secure income. Those who suffer from mental illness are even further disadvantaged by fears, inability to make decisions, and stigma. The fear of being labeled "crazy" isolates refugees further. For a psychiatric program to be successful, it must accommodate the language of refugees, respect the cultures of origin, understand the traumas and tragedies of this life, and above all have empathy for refugees.

The diverse patient population in our program includes Vietnamese, including Vietnamese Catholics and Buddhists, highly educated Vietnamese, and impoverished Vietnamese Boat People, who traveled in small boats over oceans to find safety; Cambodians, who endured the horrors of the regime of Pol Pot, a rigid Communist regent who killed or starved to death about one-third of the population from 1975 to 1979; Somalis, who lived with years of gang warfare; Russians, who suffered religious and political persecution; Bosnians, who endured the genocide inflicted by the Serbs in the former Yugoslavia; Ethiopian Oromos, who were persecuted and tortured by their own government; Iraqis, who suffered Saddam Hussein's rule and then the Iraqi War; and, now, Syrian refugees from that terrible disaster. The IPP patient population is shown in Table 6–1.

PSYCHIATRISTS

The program has eight psychiatrists, all faculty members—one full-time, and the rest part-time. Each psychiatrist has a mental health counselor with whom he or she works with the counselor's group of patients. The author has two clinics, one with Bosnians and one with Ethiopians, with each group having its own counselor. Each clinic has about 60–75 patients enrolled.

Psychiatrists are recruited for their cross-cultural interest as well as for their desire to work with difficult but interesting clinical patients. Obviously, the psychiatrists need to be tolerant, warm, and empathetic and to like working with patients from different cultures. Three psychiatrists, including the author, have worked in the clinic for almost 40 years, three other psychiatrists have worked in the clinic for over 10 years, and two others, including the IPP's medical director, are relatively new. Clinical competence, as well as the continuity of the medical staff, has enabled the program to remain stable.

The psychiatrist takes the original history, which is sometimes challenging because of issues of trust and prior severe trauma on the part of

TABLE 6–1. Patient population of the Intercultural Psychiatric Program (in 2018)

Ethnic group	n	Conflict
Vietnamese	296	Boat people, Vietnam War
Somali	135	Gang warfare
Cambodian	56	Pol Pot regime
Arabic	78	Iraqi, under Saddam Hussein's rule, and Iraq War
Farsi speaking	89	Persecution under the Iranian red guard
Bosnian	113	Genocide
Russian	70	Religious and political persecution
Mein (Hill tribe people of Laos)	29	Indo-China War
Ethiopian	50	Oromo people persecuted by own government
Nepali (from Bhutan)	30	Nepalese forcefully removed from Bhutan and sent back to Nepal
Burmese	18	Oppression against the minorities in Burma
Lao	15	Indo-China War
Syrian	3	Syrian War
Other	3	
Total	989	

Note. Approximately 60% of the patients are female. Ages range from 20 to 30 years, with median age of 40. Torture survivors officially make up 25% of the total IPP clinic population.

the patients. The diagnosis is made, and treatment is negotiated with the patient with help and explanation from the counselor. Medicine is usually prescribed; the decision to prescribe medication needs to be explained to patients, who often do not see a need for it, especially for the long term. Supportive psychotherapy and medication management are provided for long-term treatment, because the patients' conditions are often chronic. Social and legal help are often needed, and the psychiatrists frequently write letters for the patients regarding disability, asylum requests, and citizenship exemptions from English requirements.

Each psychiatrist works as a medical physician when the patient has no primary care doctor. This involves providing routine medical treatment, including managing diabetes and hypertension, giving injections, and providing medical education. Almost universally, the psychiatrist, counselor, and patient form an effective working relationship.

In the current time of brief medical appointments, we allow 60–90 minutes for the original interview with a new patient and 30 minutes for each follow-up session. Some patients take more time, and some take less, but the sessions are not to be rushed so as to maintain a respectable, calm relationship with each patient.

THE COUNSELORS

Unlike other programs, which use interpreters who may vary in skill and interest, we have a full-time staff of counselors from the patients' own ethnic group. We have found this to be the most efficient and best way to operate a multi-ethnic clinic. Each ethnic group is served by counselors from that ethnic group. The counselors are chosen for their personal characteristics of warmth and genuineness and for having respect in the community they serve, as well as for their mental health knowledge. In the case of the largest patient group, the Vietnamese, there are three counselors.

At the beginning of the program, most mental health counselors did not have college degrees but were accepted by the county and by the State Mental Health Division as professional (counselors) because of the need. Now, of the 12 current IPP counselors, 9 have master's degrees.

The counselors have multiple roles. Their primary role is as interpreters, working with the psychiatrist. Often, the counselors provide cultural information to the psychiatrist and medical information to the patient. The counselors take phone calls from the patients, which is an advantage because they speak the language and are familiar with the patient's history. The counselors also provide case management in assisting patients with their medical appointments and housing issues, and they provide individual counseling sessions, as well as group socialization experiences. About half of the patients are involved in some form of group activity. The counselors are essential in program continuity and patient engagement. To my knowledge, we are the only refugee program that is using full-time counselors as interpreters instead of on-call interpreters.

About half of the counselors have personal trauma histories, some very severe. As they interpret for the psychiatrist, the counselors can be reliving their own traumas. Support by the staff through group meetings can relieve some of this stress.

ADMINISTRATIVE STRUCTURE

The medical director of the IPP reports to the chairman of the department of psychiatry, who reports to the dean of the school of medicine. There is a supervisor of the counselors, but this supervisor reports to the medical director as well. All the counselors and administrative staff are employees of the OHSU School of Medicine. The administrative staff consists of four persons: one receptionist; two staff who are responsible for the clinic's administrative needs and for giving support to the counselors; and one medical director, who is responsible for the clinic operations and budget.

The clinic operations are funded by clinically generated revenue and grant funding. Most of the income from insurance is from Medicaid and Medicare and is necessary to meet requirements of the state Mental Health Division, which authorizes the fund. Another source of funding is the Office of Refugee Resettlement, which provides help for torture survivors who have no insurance and no other source of income. The university charges for overhead costs but provides support for legal services, human resources, electronic health records, and billing for services.

Complying with the service and documentation requirements for the state Mental Health Division generates administrative issues. The advantage to the Mental Health Division is that patients who could not be managed in the existing mental health system have access to a culturally sensitive program from which to receive ongoing care. The advantage to the medical school is that medical students and residents have an opportunity to experience the cross-cultural treatment of traumatized refugees.

RESEARCH

The program has proved to be a rich source of research material. Faculty in the program have published well over 100 papers and book chapters related to cultural psychiatry and trauma issues. We developed the Vietnamese Depression Scale (Kinzie et al. 1982); identified how a culturally sensitive clinic works (Kinzie and Manson 1983); identified PTSD in Cambodian patients (Kinzie et al. 1984) after DSM-III described the disorder; reported the high rate of hypertension and diabetes in the refugee population (Kinzie et al. 2008); reviewed how anti-adrenergic medicines reduce nightmares (Boehnlein and Kinzie 2007); outlined the elements of psychotherapy with traumatized refugees (Kinzie 2001); and described socialization group therapy with refugee patients (Kinzie et al. 1988). Outside of the clinic, we described the psychiatric disorders of Cambodian high school students and reported their outcomes (Kinzie et al. 1982; Sack et al. 1986). The program was awarded the Gold Award for Service by the American Psychiatric Association in 1988 and the Education Award by the American College of Psychiatrists in 2003.

OUTCOMES

It is difficult to do outcome studies in a busy clinic. The groups are culturally quite different in their adherence to time schedules. The Bosnian and Vietnamese patients almost always keep their appointments on time. The Cambodians tend to come all at the same time and talk among each other before and after their individual appointments. The Africans seem to be less concerned about actual appointment times, and in a typical clinic in which 8 patients are scheduled, 10 might show up, 6 of the scheduled patients and 4 who have dropped in. However, in a review of 100 patients scheduled for psychiatrist's appointments, 80% of the patients kept the appointment, a high number for a refugee psychiatric clinic, especially for often-illiterate refugees. In a prospective study of 22 severely traumatized patients followed for a year, 20 showed marked improvement, although 2 did not (Kinzie et al. 2012).

We have had very few hospitalizations of our patients. Most cases are managed through outpatient care. However, when hospitalizations are necessary, the ethnic counselors aid the process through excellent communication with the hospital staff and with the patients' family. This greatly helps the inpatient unit staff understand issues with the patients' culture, and it also helps family members understand the psychiatric treatment.

Unusual for a PTSD population, we have seen very few patients with alcohol use disorders. Also, we have had very few deaths from suicide among our patients. The best we can tell, the program has had five deaths from suicide through the 40 years it has been in operation, all of these by patients with schizophrenia. The cultural make-up of the clinic, where the majority of patients are from countries that are predominately Muslim or Buddhist, likely accounts for the reduced alcohol use and suicidal behavior.

The following case histories illustrate how the clinic works. The author was the psychiatrist involved in all the case histories, and therefore the first person will be used.

Case 1

A 68-year-old Ethiopian man with a graduate degree from Ethiopia was first seen in 2003, when he presented with marked psychiatric symptoms. He was a member of a persecuted group in Ethiopia and was tortured, including being placed in a dark, underground cell for 1 month and beaten over his head and back. At initial presentation, his symptoms included nightmares, flashbacks, irritability, poor sleep, and depression. I was involved with his patient visits every 2 months. The visits involved medicine management to control his nightmares and sleep disturbances. In addition, because most of the time he was without insurance or a primary care physician, I managed his blood pressure.

The ethnic counselor, who was from the same culture as the patient, was very involved in the case, usually seeing the patient on his own every month. Their visits involved the discussion of medicine, because the patient seemed unable to maintain consistent medical treatment. The counselor interpreted for the patient in his primary care appointments when, later, the patient was seen by his own primary care physician. The patient had many financial problems during this time due to having to lose time at work due to illness. Because of lack of income, the patient sometimes went without medicine. Also, the patient did not know how to fill out the forms necessary to obtain medical assistance. The counselor made home visits and joint visits with the patient's son to provide information about financial support. It became apparent that the patient was getting more confused at times, and the counselor helped him fill out forms for food stamps. Later in treatment, the counselor started socialization group therapy for Ethiopian patients, which provided social support for this patient. Overall, this patient's symptoms improved.

In treatment, with the involvement of both the psychiatrist and the counselor, the patient was able to obtain and take his medicine regularly. Clearly, without the counselor's availability to make home visits and help with information, this patient would have been completely disabled and isolated.

Case 2

A young Vietnamese woman presented with complaints of various somatic symptoms that did not seem to improve with any medical treatment. She related her symptoms to the death of her husband, a soldier in the Vietnamese army. One time the Vietnamese counselor was called out of the room, and the patient began to speak in fair English. The patient showed a terrible burn scar on her leg, where her husband had thrown boiling water on her. Because of multiple episodes of abuse, she was glad he had been killed, a fact she could not reveal to the female Vietnamese counselor. When the counselor returned, the patient resumed her set of somatic complaints related to symptoms. It took several more sessions for the patient to be able to reveal her anger about her deceased husband to the Vietnamese counselor.

Case 3

Some trauma stories are difficult to tell and difficult to hear. In an initial history, the patient began to describe her history of long torture. The counselor himself was a torture survivor, and when the patient began discussing the current political situation in their home country, it took some necessary effort on the part of both counselor and patient to get back to the difficult trauma history, as both were avoiding the issue. It took gentle interviewing for the patient to reveal her horrific traumas and for the counselor to feel support in the interview and in debriefing with the psychiatric team later.

Case 4

Cambodians had a very traumatic and tragic history under Pol Pot. It requires a great deal of patience in taking the history to get even the outline of what happened. This interview with a Cambodian patient was done with an experienced Cambodian counselor, with a Cambodian trainee observing. During the interview, I realized that the trainee had picked up a magazine and had started to read it. It was pointed out to him that he needed to pay attention to the patient. Later it was discovered that the trainee had suffered under Pol Pot and had had family members killed. He was reliving his own traumas in a painful way, which he was trying to avoid.

Case 5

The Bosnian War provided some of the most inhumane examples of human cruelty ever. The patient, an elderly Bosnian man, had experienced severe trauma in a concentration camp where friends were killed. He was saved when a Serbian officer recognized him and drove him to the edge of town. It was only after several years of treatment that he revealed what he went through. A particularly upsetting event he had witnessed was when he and other Bosnians were separated and were not given food. Finally, a guard gave food to one of the prisoners, who gulped it down, not giving any to his own son. Later he told of the worst event he had seen. He was forced to clean a house with bodies of Bosnians, who had been murdered to make room for the Serbs. From a pile of bodies came out a beautiful, probably 3-year-old blond girl with her hands up crying. The patient picked up the girl and took her to the guard and asked what should be done. The guard picked up the girl and threw her against a tree and killed her. There was nothing to say. The Bosnian counselor began to shed tears. Sadness overwhelmed all three. Despite the brutality, the patient seemed relieved to finally talk about it.

CONCLUSION

The Oregon Model providing psychiatric care to refugees using highly trained ethnic counselors has been highly successful in treatment and sustainable for 40 years. As far as we know, no other program has used this model. Why is this?

The reasons seem to vary. One reason is that it is difficult to get psychiatrists involved in terms of interest and expenses. Another issue is that it is hard to find trained ethnic counselors. A third issue is that many programs are psychotherapy based with reliance on therapists with interpreters. Such programs may often ignore major mental illness needs and deal only with psychological issues. Many programs rely on grants and donations to keep the programs functioning, and reliance on such funding sources makes sustainability very difficult. Indeed, many refugee programs have closed because of financial problems.

Aspiring refugee programs should consider becoming a mental health program approved by the state Mental Health Division in order to receive Medicaid and Medicare funds. This step requires medical staffing and compliance with rules regarding staffing, records, and quality assurance. Many refugee programs' directors and staff have said that the time and expense to get started are too difficult to even attempt.

We have shown it can be done, admittedly with much administrative effort. We hope others will follow this model or some aspects of it to help more refugees receive needed help.

KEY CLINICAL POINTS

- The Oregon Intercultural Psychiatric Program (IPP) has been in existence for over 40 years treating refugees and asylum seekers.

- Its longevity has been dependent on faculty psychiatrists, the majority of whom have stayed with the program for at least 15 years.

- The critical part of the clinic is that it uses full-time counselor-interpreters from the patients' own cultures. The counselors act as interpreters with the psychiatrist, but as case managers and socialization group therapists when they are working with the patient on their own. Therefore, patients always have a person with them who knows them. In addition, a staff member who understands the patient's language is also available if there is a need for the patient to call the clinic.

- The psychiatrist provides evaluation, psychotherapy (usually supportive), medication management, and letters of support for receiving government medical assistance or citizenship application.

- Being a part of a medical school provides a firm administration structure and clear lines of authority.

- Having Medicare, Medicaid, and help from the Office of Refugee Resettlement provides financial security.

- A long-term program such as the IPP provides a patient base for research, especially of long-term clinical outcomes.

REFERENCES

Boehnlein JK, Kinzie JD: Pharmacologic reduction of CNS noradrenergic activity in PTSD: the case for clonidine and prazosin. J Psychiatr Pract 13(2):72–78, 2007 17414682

Kinzie JD: Psychotherapy for massively traumatized refugees: the therapist variable. Am J Psychother 55(4):475–490, 2001 11824215

Kinzie JD, Manson SM: Five-years' experience with Indochinese refugee patients. Journal of Operational Psychiatry 14(2):105–111, 1983

Kinzie JD, Tran KA, Breckenridge A, et al: An Indochinese refugee psychiatric clinic: culturally accepted treatment approaches. Am J Psychiatry 137(11):1429–1432, 1980 7435679

Kinzie JD, Manson SM, Vinh DT, et al: Development and validation of a Vietnamese-language depression rating scale. Am J Psychiatry 139(10):1276–1281, 1982 7124979

Kinzie JD, Fredrickson RH, Ben R, et al: Posttraumatic stress disorder among survivors of Cambodian concentration camps. Am J Psychiatry 141(5):645–650, 1984 6711684

Kinzie JD, Leung P, Bui A, et al: Group therapy with Southeast Asian refugees. Community Ment Health J 24(2):157–166, 1988 3402200

Kinzie JD, Riley C, McFarland B, et al: High prevalence rates of diabetes and hypertension among refugee psychiatric patients. J Nerv Ment Dis 196(2):108–112, 2008 18277218

Kinzie JD, Kinzie JM, Sedighi B, et al: Prospective one-year treatment outcomes of tortured refugees: a psychiatric approach. Torture 22(1):1–10, 2012 23086001

Sack WH, Angell RH, Kinzie JD, et al: The psychiatric effects of massive trauma on Cambodian children II. The family, the home, and the school. J Am Acad Child Adolesc Psychiatry 25(3):377–383, 1986

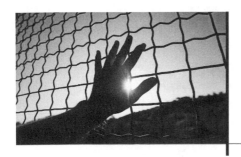

Chapter 7

CHILDREN AND ADOLESCENTS

Keith Cheng, M.D.
Paria Zarrinnegar, M.D.

It is estimated by the United Nations that worldwide there are 10 million refugee children below the age of 18 years (United Nations High Commission for Refugees 2017). Youth who move with or without their families to escape persecution, war, or other types of violence typically experience high levels of stress prior, during, and after moving from their homes to another country. Refugee youth may be leaving their home country because of devastating violence such as torture, loss of loved ones to murder, loss of a home to bombing, and/or sexual assault by terrorists or even neighbors. Many families leave their homes for refugee camps to escape capture by soldiers or rebels who treat civilians without any regard for their well-being. These stresses prior to leaving a home country are frequently replaced with the horrors of living in refugee camps, where there are new stresses. Lack of food and adequate housing, basic services such as running water and sewage management, and security are sometimes more stressful than the reasons for leaving home.

Infectious diseases, sexual assaults, and no access to medical care are often the norm in many of these camps. If a child and his or her family are lucky enough to be transferred from a refugee camp to a first-world country, they are beset with a new set of challenges. New language, unfamiliar food, disapproving neighbors, and unaccommodating schools are all challenges immigrant youth have to face. Furthermore, with changes in public opinion and ever-changing political policy, governmental responses are frequently chaotic. These responses can traumatize children with results that are as devastating as those from armed political conflict and displacement to refugee camps. Some governments will separate refugee children, including infants, from their parents as a strategy to halt the influx of refugees. In some countries there are cases in which children are left in detention facilities when their parents are deported. Immigration authorities may not know how to reconnect these deported parents and their children. The children of these deported parents may languish in detention centers in a foreign country with no idea whether they will see their parents again. So, at every stage of the immigration process, refugee youth are at risk for catastrophic trauma. Clinical experience reveals that the majority of refugee youth are lucky not to have experienced multiple traumatic events.

THE CHALLENGE

Clinicians working with refugee populations face a number of obstacles. There is a dearth of research that can guide clinicians. Most interventions for traumatized youth are developed on the basis of research conducted in European or American subjects. Psychotherapies that are based on a patient's ability to describe his or her feeling states (e.g., cognitive-behavioral therapy [CBT]) require facility with language. Immigrant youth are frequently not facile with a new language in a new country. Furthermore, open expression of feelings may not be considered appropriate in their culture of origin. Immigrant parents may feel threatened by traditional family therapy and may need nontraditional engagement strategies. These parents may be overwhelmed by their own traumatic events and need treatment before they are able to participate in family work. Even biological treatments, which are not considered bound by culture, need to consider ethnogenomic factors. Medication doses that are effective in Caucasian populations may not be effective in certain ethnic groups. Ethnic differences in liver function are known to make the usual medication dose recommendations either too high or too low for certain populations. Furthermore, in research on medication adherence, nonwhite patients have been found to be more likely to have lower adherence (Lanouette et al. 2009). It is not uncommon for immigrant parents to take prescriptions for their child from psychiatric appointments and never fill them.

Immigrant refugee youth are at a higher risk for sustaining multiple psychological traumas and for developing psychopathology. Treating clinicians, therefore, are tasked with cases in which comorbid diagnoses are the norm rather than the exception. Also, the ability to recover is hindered by multiple traumas that take place in a context of displacement from home. In a study with 30-month follow-up, PTSD, depression, and somatic complaints decreased with time in internally displaced children, but psychosocial adaptation remained worse in these children and did not improve with time (Fazel et al. 2012; Powell and Durakovic-Belko 2000). Direct exposure to violence and adverse events is associated with an increased likelihood of psychological dysfunction in refugee children. There are studies that show the development of PTSD is related to personal traumatic experiences, and particularly those traumas that occurred away from home. Youth who directly experienced traumatic events showed increased levels of anxiety and sleep disturbances compared with youth who did not experience such events (Hjern et al. 1991).

Working with youth from immigrant families presents treating clinicians with a multitude of cultural challenges. These challenges can include community attitudes toward immigrants, immigrant attitudes about parenting, and immigrant youth attitudes about living in a new place. As with their parents, immigrant youth are confronted with the existing socioeconomic culture of the community into which they have moved. The hosting communities may be filled with individuals who are xenophobic. A new person or his or her family is feared and hated, before any interaction has occurred. These challenges often present barriers to assessment and treatment.

OVERVIEW OF WORKING WITH REFUGEE CHILDREN AND FAMILIES

WORKING WITH PARENTS

The key to working with refugee children is to establish a good working relationship with their parents. Parents who do not feel connected to treating clinicians will not bring their children in for treatment, particularly if they had a negative experience during the assessment appointment. Parents are frequently suspicious of medical or psychiatric clinicians.

They are afraid they will be exposed as bad or abusive and have their children taken away. Feeling inadequate for having children with behavioral problems can be shaming. Coming to strangers who may not understand their culture, they fear disapproval. Therefore, clinicians need to be careful about their attitudes toward different cultures. They should seek to understand refugee children and their families from a mindset of "What happened to this child and his family?" rather than "What is wrong with this child and his family?" Validating the positive aspects of the home culture can often dispel the fear of being misunderstood. Parents are often befuddled by the new reality of parenting a child in a different culture. Helping refugee parents understand the challenges of raising children in a new culture will clarify what work needs to be done. If they understand these challenges, they will better understand treatment recommendations and how to implement them.

Emphasizing transcultural norms can lessen that feeling of being alone in a new place. Clinician and parental goals can be the same. Aiming for children to have healthy relationships with their parents, to be successful in school, and to get along with new peers is a universal goal for both immigrant parents and their new communities. A nonjudgmental review of pros and cons of rigid adherence to parenting styles of the culture of origin can be illuminating for refugee parents. With this review they can better understand why their child may be rebelling against what they would consider a regular request to be compliant with their family norms.

Experienced therapists know that seeking an intercultural compromise is the gold standard for family work with immigrant parents and their children. The delicate process of identifying the best of both cultures and adopting them as goals for healthy adaptation is the foundation for successful parental guidance and counseling. The Collaborative Problem Solving (CPS) principle of communicating in a way the listener can tolerate is a good example of how to engage refugee parents (Think:Kids 2019). Clinicians who are sensitive to how they communicate to refugee parents will be more successful in engaging them to keep their child in treatment. Using CPS principles can also be an effective way for immigrant parents to decrease conflict with their children who are trying to fit into a new culture and peer group. Modeling CPS principles can be good for both treatment engagement and treatment planning.

WORKING WITH REFUGEE CHILDREN

As with parents, validating a refugee youth's feelings about being in a new place, the difficulties of fitting in with a new peer group, and contending with parental conflict is the most important key to working with immigrant children. Trusting adults in a new place can be a complicated process. Refugee youth are often intimidated by therapists and doctors; they are afraid of new relationships and of being misunderstood. Fortunately, most refugee youths respond to a good listener who can understand their situation. Although building trust can be easy, keeping that trust is more challenging. In particular, clinicians should strive to understand the impact of dual-language competence on a child's adaptation and functioning. Identifying impediments in language acquisition will help inform the quality of assessment data obtained and how the child is likely to cope in the school setting. A refugee's likelihood of having a successful transition is tied to his or her ability to communicate with treating clinicians, peers, and school staff. In the assessment phase, clinicians should make sure they conduct the evaluation in the language that both the child and parents are proficient. Lack of appropriate interpretation services can lead to inaccurate diagnoses and adverse clinical outcomes (Flores et al. 2003).

For adolescents and mature school-age children, the initial clinical interview can be a rich source of assessment data. Clinicians should take the time to elicit the perceived age-related cultural expectations for school, home, and peer relationships. They should examine for possible cultural divergences and whether these conflicts play a role in the reason the child has come for treatment. Peer group interactions are important to immigrant youth, and questions about ethnicity, religious identity, racism, or gender issues should be included in the interview following the child's lead. Some children will not be able to answer all the pertinent questions for the assessment. So, clinicians should be able to select and adapt their questions to ensure that they are culturally sensitive and developmentally appropriate. In general, the younger the refugee youth, the less likely he or she is able to provide accurate socioeconomic questions about the family. Therefore, these questions should usually be reserved for parents. DSM-5 provides a comprehensive set of assessment questions to obtain an accurate cross-cultural history (American Psychiatric Association 2013). Clinicians new to providing assessments of refugee youth will find them helpful in structuring their assessment interviews.

WORKING WITH PARENTS AND CHILDREN ON IDENTIFICATION ISSUES

Treating refugee youth in isolation from their family is likely to be less successful. It is important to meet with a child and his or her family as part of any treatment, particularly in cases in which there is a high degree of conflict around acculturation issues. Although there are varying differences in a child's desire to assimilate into a new culture, most immigrant youth will experience some friction with their parents around what is allowable behavior. These rub points usually revolve around the conflict between home-of-origin values and new country and community cultures. Andrew Solomon, in his book *Far from the Tree*, describes the conflict that arises from parental desire for "vertical identity" and a child's desire for "horizontal identity" (Solomon 2013). Although he does not specifically address how this applies to immigrant families, this concept works well to describe the conflict that refugee children experience with their parents. Vertical identity consists of attitudes and values that are passed from one generation to another. Horizontal identity arises when internal or external differences arise from new or unexpected situations, like living in a new country. For immigrant and refugee youth there is a natural pathway to a new intense horizontal identity. In order to survive in a new social setting, immigrant youths usually try to fit in with the dominant peer group. Adopting the dominant culture social customs and attitudes helps decrease the amount foreignness that prevents acceptance by the new set of peers.

This of course leads to a horizontal identity that frequently becomes in conflict with parental wishes for their child to have a dominant vertical identity, retaining the values and culture of the home country. Describing these identity processes and how they can lead to conflict can be a difficult task. Explanations in a language foreign to parents is just another barrier to understanding these concepts. Helping immigrant parents and their children understand these identity pathways can be facilitated by using a graphic aid like a pie chart. Parents can diagram in a pie chart what percentage of the home country traditions and culture they prefer to use in parenting, in contrast to using the new country parenting styles. Children can draw a pie chart that depicts which parental style they would like their parents to use (i.e., home country vs. new country). This visual aid can rapidly lead to an understanding of vertical and horizontal identity conflict.

Visual aids like a pie chart can be used as "cross-cultural comparison tools" in therapy sessions with great effect. Immigrant youths will develop horizontal identifications that are not shared with their parents. Their parents will often have a strong reaction to those identities that are in contrast to the vertical identifications they want for their children. Although each family resolves these conflicts in its own way, ultimately parental acceptance and even acceptance of some of the horizontal identity will help smooth their children's adaptation to their new home country. Hence, using the metaphor of adopting the best parts of two cultures, vertical and horizontal identities, can lead to healthy intercultural compromise.

BEING A LIAISON BETWEEN REFUGEE FAMILIES AND SCHOOLS AND OTHER COMMUNITY AGENCIES

Refugee youth and their families will often be connected with schools and community agencies. Because all children need to be in an educational setting, clinicians will frequently have to be in contact with schoolteachers and school administrators to help schools understand what special needs a student may have. Refugee children will frequently need "English as a second language" classes. Immigrant youth often display behaviors that are normal for living in a third-world country or refugee camp that are inappropriate for traditional school settings. Parental involvement in the school setting can be confusing for immigrant parents. Teachers need to understand the circumstances of refugee families and how their life experiences may create hindrances to usual family involvement. Immigrant parents are often unable to assist their children with homework or other tasks requested of them. Clinician contact to provide "refugee psychosocial education" for teachers and school administrators usually helps to pave the way for easier transitions into academic settings. Schools appreciate a behavioral support services that clinicians can provide when refugee youth display difficult behaviors that school staff are unable to manage.

Child protective services are frequently involved with refugee families. Many clinicians who have worked with refugee families have the experience of addressing the challenge of corporal punishment. This parental style of discipline can be the source of children being removed from biological parents by social services, even when removal is detrimental to the youth. Some immigrant children will use child protective services abuse reporting to avoid discipline at home. Most of the time social service agencies will welcome or seek input from clinicians when these agencies are called on to assess abuse or neglect situations. Sometimes, however, they will not contact treating clinicians and will make decisions without having the full picture. In these cases, clinicians may have to insert themselves into investigative process and provide uninvited information for the best interest of the child. Stereotyping is common when a dominant culture is in charge of assessment of immigrants. There is a body of research that shows that well-meaning people who are not overtly biased and do not believe they are prejudiced typically demonstrate implicit negative racial attitudes and stereotypes (Dovidio et al. 1996).

In the unfortunate situation when a refugee youth is placed in a juvenile or immigration detention center, treating clinicians may be the only resource for the families to rely on to negotiate these complex worlds. Detention staff with little or no clinical training will depend on treating clinicians to help them understand special needs of their detainees. They will frequently request specific treatment recommendations for refugee youth when an identified treating clinician becomes identified. Clinicians should not feel they need to wait to be asked before contacting these agencies. Detention staff need a clinical point of view and will often welcome this perspective.

Refugee youth and families may also rely on clinicians to serve as liaisons to physical health needs as well as other specialty services such as occupational or physical therapy. Housing and other social service needs should be part of a review of systems for clinicians. Referral information for these services should be available to support refugee children and their families.

Case 1: Changing Nationality

Alia is a 10-year-old Afghani female brought in for evaluation of intense anxiety following a motor vehicle accident. A month prior to evaluation, she and her mother were hit by a car while in a crosswalk. They did not sustain significant physical or neurological injuries from the accident. For the past month Alia had been struggling with frequent stomachaches, excessive sweating, low appetite, hypervigilance, and intrusive memories of the car accident. She had not been able to sleep by herself since the accident. She was plagued by nightmares most nights. She was afraid to leave the house. During the evaluation, it was revealed that Alia had been experiencing similar symptoms for the past 2 years and that these symptoms had intensified since her collision with the car. She had been evaluated for her somatic symptoms and medical causes had been ruled out.

Alia's family was from Afghanistan. She, along with her mother and three older brothers, came to the United States a year prior as refugees after spending over a year in a refugee camp in Pakistan. They left their country after Alia's father, a physician, was killed by the Taliban when she was 6 years old. Alia was exposed to war and combat in her hometown. On arrival to the United States, Alia started school, where she was academically successful and considered one of the best students in her class. Alia had several friends at school but was repeatedly harassed by other children there after they found out she was from Afghanistan. They said she was a member of the "Taliban." Alia reported feeling confused and overwhelmed by these incidents. The thought of being associated with a group of people who had murdered her father was overwhelming at times. In a group therapy session Alia revealed that in order to avoid being teased about being a member of the Taliban, she changed her Muslim name to a Western name and told school peers she was from India.

Despite Alia's supportive family, her superior intellectual abilities, and desire to improve her function, she continued to struggle with significant worries and avoidant behaviors over her initial course of treatment. She would avoid riding in the family car, taxi cabs, or public transportation. She continued to insist on sleeping with her mother. Trials of selective serotonin reuptake inhibitors and trauma-focused CBT were only partially effective. After the clinician discussed these issues with Alia in a family therapy session, it became apparent that a sense of loneliness and being constantly bullied at school had a huge impact on Alia's emotional health. Alia and her family decided to change her school. Alia found her new school environment more accepting of her ethnic background. She eventually found some new friends and went back to using her given name. She gradually began to feel more comfortable spending time outside of the home and eventually was able to travel in the family car without intense anxiety.

This case of a youth with severe PTSD shows how trauma plays a significant role in the ongoing presence of debilitating symptoms. Alia suffered multiple psychological traumas before, during, and after immigration to a new home country. She was not able to fully recover, however, until she was removed from the trauma trigger of daily bullying at school. Schools can be a stabilizing feature in the unsettled lives of refugee students; they can provide safe spaces for new encounters, interactions, and learning opportunities (Matthews 2008). In the best-case scenario, schools can provide a safe holding environment where traumatized youth can move from trauma reenactments to determining new adaptive narratives. New schools, however, can also be a source of trauma to refugee youths. Mental health providers should be vigilant about bullying that can occur in school settings. Moreover, clinicians should focus not only on the interventions that take place in the office. Frequently, solutions may be environmental rather than rooted in the traditional approaches of psychotherapy and psychotropic medications.

Case 2: Xenophobia

Hana, daughter of an Iraqi family, first was referred to our clinic at age 12 from her middle school for psychiatric evaluation. The chief complaints included difficulty sustaining attention and following directions and disruptive behaviors (e.g., intimidating other kids, lying, leaving class without permission) that had resulted in three suspensions in the first 3 months of the academic year. During initial evaluation, Hana and her parents reported symptoms consistent with ADHD, as well as depression. Hana's family had moved to the United States from Iraq 10 years prior as refugees. She lived with both parents and four siblings. Her father was the only financial provider, and her mother was the main parent supervising the children. Hana was mostly brought up as an American child and voiced a desire to be more American as she entered adolescence. Her parents often felt confused about nuances of Western culture but hoped that their children could blend in the culture of their Muslim home. Her mother voiced difficulties setting any behavioral limits for Hana. There was no history of significant psychological trauma or medical issues.

During her initial assessment appointment, she was diagnosed with ADHD, oppositional defiant disorder, and mild depression. She was treated with stimulants along with individual and family therapy during a 3-year period and showed enough improvement that her parents felt that Hana no longer needed treatment. Her parents were advised to return to clinic as needed.

Three years later Hana's parents made an appointment for Hana. However, she did not return with her parents. She had recently alleged that her biological parents were physically abusing her. Child protective services completed an assessment and decided to place her in a foster home. The allegations had happened in the context of increasing oppositional behavior and rule-breaking behavior, including running away from home. She wanted to live with a new boyfriend, so she told the police that she was being abused. Child protective services never contacted her mental health clinicians. In the foster care placement, she continued to show conduct-disordered behaviors such as drinking and leaving the house without permission, leaving the school grounds during class, and destroying public property at a park, and she engaged in multiple unprotected sexual encounters. It appeared to her outpatient team that she may be suffering from a manic episode. After several attempts to contact her state-appointed guardian, her family therapist attended a team meeting to discuss the need for psychiatric reassessment and possible reconciliation for Hana and her family. However, this request was rebuffed. "She is misbehaving because she was abused. We can't return this child to this Iraqi family; they will abuse her again."

Hana was returned to the custody of her biological parents because social services ran out of placements. Hana may have been showing early signs of developing bipolar disorder when she was first assessed at age 12 years. By the time she was placed in state custody, Hana was in the midst of a bipolar mania, too symptomatic to be safely placed in any foster or group home placement. With assistance of her outpatient team, she was placed in a psychiatric residential program, where she was formally diagnosed with bipolar disorder type 1, in a manic episode. When stabilized, Hana admitted that her boyfriend had suggested that she should accuse her parents of abuse so she could escape their custody. Her parents were actually quite liberal and supported Hana's wish to identify primarily as an American youth. Instead of adopting the best American culture, Hana, in the throes of mania, engaged in a self-destructive world of drugs and delinquent behaviors. It is not entirely clear whether Hana would have received needed treatment sooner if social services had contacted her outpatient providers at the time she came into state care. But it is clear that her state-appointed guardian showed considerable signs of prejudice to Muslim parents and culture. In the medical world evidence exists that provider biases adversely affect quality of care for minority patients. Research does suggest that mental health providers are influenced by their feelings about race and ethnic groups. In a study of mental health clinicians, those "primed" with African American stereotype–laden descriptions were more likely to assess a hypothetical patient negatively than those primed with neutral descriptions (Pumariega et al. 2013).

Case 3: A Monk Instead of Medications

David, a 15-year-old who lived with his immigrant Vietnamese parents, was referred for outpatient follow-up after inpatient psychiatric hospitalization for an initial manic episode with psychotic features. He had been experiencing auditory hallucination, mood dysregulation, and a significant decline in his academic function for the several months prior to hospitalization. While in the hospital, he was started on antipsychotics and his condition was partially stabilized.

David had no history of prior psychiatric or medical problems. His birth history and developmental history were unremarkable. He had been a straight-A student until his sophomore year. There was no history of substance use or traumatic experiences or known history of mental illness in the family. David's parents moved from Vietnam to a new country before David was born as refugees. The family actively practiced Buddhism. Six months after the initial manic episode, his mother reported that she had stopped David's medications because he seemed to be back to his old self. He went back to passing all classes and stayed in remission for the rest of the academic year. The following summer, however, David presented with symptoms of depression, including lethargy, isolation, and significant psychomotor retardation. His parents were worried about his lack of motivation. David's treating clinician reinitiated medications and provided extensive psychoeducation about the course of bipolar disorder. David's parents, however, were not convinced that the current presentation was related to "bipolar disorder" and that medications could help. He did not look manic. He had no energy. They believed that David would benefit most from a healing power from their religion to help him regain his energy and purify his soul. David, himself, was ambivalent about medication, but he did not believe in healing powers. Contact was made with the family's local Buddhist monk to see if a collaboration was possible. Fortunately, the Buddhist clergyman did not find a reason to recommend against taking medication for a "medical" illness. With the support of the monk, David agreed to medications. David's psychotropic medications were restarted, and he was able to recover enough to get back to school.

For David, it was fortunate that a monk from his temple was in support of medical treatments. If a patient's family participates in organized religious activities, clinicians should consider consulting and collaborating with the traditional healers and leaders of their chosen faith. Collaboration with indigenous traditional healers and church clergy can ameliorate cultural loyalty conflicts within families and children. These partnerships may also improve access to care in populations unfamiliar with or even mistrusting of the medical or psychiatric model. This is typically feasible when traditional healing methods complement or enhance and do not directly conflict with the efficacy of allopathic psychotropic treatments. Many traditional healers are often reticent to identify themselves as collaborating with Western-trained clinicians. However, mutual respect and education in exchanging information and perspectives can foster collaboration (Pumariega et al. 2013).

Case 4: Second-Language Concerns

Faria, a 7-year-old Somali second-grader, was referred by her school for evaluation of disruptive behaviors and poor academic performance. Her family reported that Faria had had behavioral problems for the past year since enrolling in a new school. At school, she had a short attention span, often struggled to stay seated in the classroom, and appeared to be driven by a motor. She also had difficulty completing schoolwork, especially when it came to reading or language activities, which was assumed to be due to language barriers by school. The school staff communicated with Faria's parents that she should be evaluated for possible ADHD. Her parents had left Somalia before she was conceived, and she was born in a refugee camp in Kenya following a noncomplicated pregnancy. She had no significant previous medical or psychiatric history.

In the clinic, she was noted to be fidgety and physically hyperactive, walking around the room many times. On mental status exam, Faria found it difficult to answer traditional interview questions. When she did, she was very soft spoken and would only speak in short phrases. Interestingly, her parents reported she would only speak English at home and not in their ethnic language. Faria was not able to spell her last name. Further testing showed she had a significant language dysfunction. With the provisional diagnostic impression of ADHD and learning disorder, she was referred for further testing, which confirmed a diagnosis of dyslexia. Findings were communicated with school, and an Individualized Education Program (IEP) was developed for her learning disorder and ADHD. She received medication management and social skills training. Her family reported improvement in her attention span and behavioral issues at home.

It is easy to presume that an immigrant child who does not do well in a new school is having difficulty adapting to a new language. This presumption, however, is sometimes inaccurate. Faria's case demonstrates that not every refugee immigrant youth who struggles in school has problems learning a new language. In fact, if the teacher had asked Faria's mother about how Faria's brothers and sisters had adapted to a new language, she would have found out that Faria was the only child in the family struggling in school. All her siblings were doing well academically. Faria's teacher was making assumptions about her ability without important data. Thus, it is critical for teachers and clinicians to make sure they communicate with parents with an interpreter whenever there is a concern about parental language facility. Interpreters should have proper training in both the skill of interpretation and the content area being discussed. They should serve as integral members of the clinical team, function as cultural consultants when they have an understanding of the family's culture, and interpret all of the verbal, nonverbal, and implicit communications from the child and family rather than provide summaries (Pumariega et al. 2013). After an IEP evaluation for learning disabilities, Faria was identified with having dyslexia. This learning disorder qualified her for extra services. With extra support, Faria was more successful academically and less disruptive at school.

There is evidence that maintaining the first (home) language is important in accessing family and community protective factors and other benefits. Despite this evidence, there has been a poorly substantiated practice of recommending to parents that they discontinue speaking the home language to a child who is facing language, cognitive, or other academic delays. This practice has little or no empirical support, and the limited research conducted in this area suggests that children with language impairment can healthily learn two languages with no significant detrimental effects. Although it may be true that certain children with linguistic or other deficits may become overwhelmed by the additional cognitive and linguistic demands of dual language learning, recommendations to discontinue learning the home language may have potentially

serious consequences and should not be made lightly. Rather, such decisions should ideally involve full assessment by a speech-language pa-
thologist. With appropriate expertise, and consultation with the parents
and others who know the child well, an informed decision process can
be completed for the child's parents (Toppelberg and Collins 2010).

Case 5: ADHD or PTSD?

Batal, an 11-year-old Pakistani boy, was brought in for assessment by
his parents because of concerns about behavioral issues. The parents reported that these issues were mainly present at school and not at home.
Issues included difficulty remaining in the classroom and completing his
work, following directions, and poor frustration tolerance. Educational
testing had not revealed learning problems, and the school recommended ADHD evaluation. On further questioning, parents also reported that Batal had been struggling with poor sleep since a very young
age, having difficulty falling asleep and multiple nighttime awakenings.

Batal's family moved from Pakistan to the United States 4 years
prior as war refugees. When asked about their life back in their home
country, they described having a good life before war began. His parents
both held bachelor's degrees and were working as teachers. Batal's grand-
father had been killed by a local terrorist group. They reported that
Batal had not witnessed this event, but both parents were experiencing
intrusive memories and subsequent hyperarousal symptoms associated
with these traumatic experiences. They had never sought treatment for
their symptoms and had decided to move on with their lives after their
move to the United States.

When asked about Batal's trauma history, they said Batal was too
young to be affected by the trauma and immigration experience. They,
however, remembered that Batal was injured at age 4 when a bomb hit
a nearby house. Batal was playing in the kitchen next to his mother, who
was boiling water when the explosion happened. Batal sustained a burn
injury from the boiling water, and some metal shrapnel pierced his thigh.
His parents were not sure how much Batal remembered of these events,
and they avoided conversation about their life back in Pakistan in front
of him. When asked about scary memories, Batal spoke about bad people trying to invade the house. He added quickly, though, that he missed
his friends back in his home country.

In children it is not uncommon for PTSD to be mistaken for ADHD
(Kaminer et al. 2005). Batal was diagnosed provisionally with PTSD.
He was started on a low dose of clonidine. Treatment involved family
psychoeducation about trauma and PTSD symptoms. His parents began receiving treatment for their own PTSD symptoms and felt a significant improvement as a result. As Batal's PTSD responded well to

these interventions, he started to struggle with feelings of depression. So, he was engaged in weekly psychotherapy sessions to help him understand some unresolved grief issues. By the following year, he was excelling as a student in the classroom and had made many new friends. Young refugees often develop a fantasized mental image of what was left behind because they have not gained the object constancy of people, pets, and things lost in this process. They develop an understanding of the traumatic event according to their developmental stage and phase-specific ego functions and their relationship with important others involved in the traumatic event. Younger children cannot mourn as adults do. The premigration disruption of the mother-child relationship, and his mother's postmigration emotional well-being, also played a major role in how Batal experienced his immigrant experience (Volkan 2018).

Case 6: Dressing Like Britney Spears

Malika, who preferred her common Western name in place of her given Muslim name, is a 17-year old teenager who was referred for evaluation of school refusal and family conflict. Her parents reported that about a year prior, she bleached her hair without permission and started wearing provocative Western clothing. She was noted by classmates to be dressing like a famous pop icon. When she was teased for it, she got into fights with the teasing students and refused to return to school. Malika pined to be like other kids at school, but she had no friends there and often felt lonely. Her parents worried that if Malika continued to be influenced by Western culture, she would leave home prematurely before finishing school.

Malika's parents came to the United States as refugees when she was a toddler. Both parents had witnessed war in their home country but denied that Malika had been exposed to any trauma, as they had escaped to a neighbor country before she was born. Her father, who had a college degree from his home country, had been working as a janitor since arrival in the United States and suffered from depression. Her mother spoke very little English and struggled with OCD and PTSD symptoms.

Following the initial assessment, which focused mainly on family conflicts, Malika and her family did not come back for treatment until 4 years later. At that time Malika presented with complaints of "not feeling normal." She reported a 4-month history of symmetry preoccupations and fear of germs. Associated symptoms included long showers, daily multiple change of clothing, and an inability to use public restrooms. These symptoms were distressing to Malika and were impairing her ability to function. She was specifically worried that her symptoms resembled those of her mother, with whom she had ongoing conflicts. Malika was still living with her parents, who often criticized her sexually provocative attire and drug-using friends. Malika disclosed she had been raped multiple times over the prior year by different American boys. She gave a history of intermittent alcohol and cannabis use. Malika was advised to start medication to help with OCD symptoms and to engage in psychotherapy for CBT with exposure and response prevention. She struggled with medication adherence and coming to her appointments and dropped out of treatment four times. She obtained a GED degree but has never been able to live independently or get a job. She continues to feel conflicted in her relationships with her family and friends, about Western culture and her own identity.

Malika's story shows what can happen when an immigrant youth and parents are unable to find adaptive responses to cross-cultural conflicts. Acculturation has a direct impact on the developmental task of identity, just as racial/ethnic identity constitutes a significant aspect of psychological identity. Peers and family members serve as "mirrors" in which the self is reflected. For racially/ethnically diverse children and youth, this mirroring comes from two sources—the traditional cultural environment of the home and the mainstream cultural environment of peers, school, and the broader community—and conflicting images can result. Diverse children and youth often face significant pressures to assimilate into mainstream society through media images and implicit threats of social and economic marginalization. In the process of acculturation, the best adaptational outcomes are associated with the development of a bicultural identity, in which immigrant youth remain rooted in their culture of origin (often mediated by learning the home language) but have the necessary knowledge and interpersonal skills to successfully navigate mainstream culture (Pumariega and Rothe 2010; Rothe et al. 2010).

KEY POINTS

- Many refugee children have been severely traumatized, but interventions for traumatized children are typically based on Western children and may not be appropriate for refugee children.

- The key in working with refugee children is a good working relationship their parents, who may feel suspicious of the motives of the psychiatrist.

- Refugee children need to have their feelings validated, including those related to being in a new place, difficulty fitting in, and contending with parental conflicts. It is important to examine age-related cultural expectations for school, home, and peer relationships on the part of both the child and the parent.

- It is important to meet with the child and family as part of treatment, particularly when there is conflict around acculturation.

- Because the children will be in educational settings, the psychiatrist will need to be in contact with schoolteachers and administration staff to help the school understand the special needs the refugee child may feel.

- When refugee youth are placed in a detention center, the psychiatrist may be the only resource the family has to help them negotiate these complex issues.

- Severe PTSD plays a significant role in ongoing debilitating symptoms for refugee children. Also, PTSD can be mistaken for ADHD.

- The best adaptational outcomes are associated with bicultural identity by which the youth are rooted in their own culture of origin but have the necessary skills to navigate the mainstream culture.

REFERENCES

American Psychiatric Association: Diagnostic and Statistical Manual of Mental Disorders, 5th Edition. Arlington, VA, American Psychiatric Association, 2013, pp 10–11

Dovidio J, Brigham J, Johnson B, et al: Stereotyping, prejudice, and discrimination: another look, in Stereotypes and Stereotyping. Edited by Macrae CN, Stangor C, Hewstone M. New York, Guilford, 1996, pp 276–322

Fazel M, Reed RV, Panter-Brick C, Stein A: Mental health of displaced and refugee children resettled in high-income countries: risk and protective factors. Lancet 379(9812):266–282, 2012 21835459

Flores G, Laws MB, Mayo SJ, et al: Errors in medical interpretation and their potential clinical consequences in pediatric encounters. Pediatrics 111(1):6–14, 2003 12509547

Hjern A, Angel B, Höjer B: Persecution and behavior: a report of refugee children from Chile. Child Abuse Negl 15(3):239–248, 1991 2043975

Kaminer D, Seedat S, Stein DJ: Post-traumatic stress disorder in children. World Psychiatry 4(2):121–125, 2005 16633528

Lanouette NM, Folsom DP, Sciolla A, Jeste DV: Psychotropic medication nonadherence among United States Latinos: a comprehensive literature review. Psychiatr Serv 60(2):157–174, 2009 19176409

Matthews J: Schooling and settlement: refugee education in Australia. International Studies in Sociology of Education 18(1):31–45, 2008

Powell S, Durakovic-Belko E: Sarajevo 2000: the psychosocial consequences of war. Results of empirical research from the territory of former Yugoslavia. Presented at a symposium held at the Faculty of Philosophy at Sarajevo, July 7–8, 2000

Pumariega AJ, Rothe E: Leaving no children or families outside: the challenges of immigration. Am J Orthopsychiatry 80(4):505–515, 2010 20950291

Pumariega AJ, Rothe E, Mian A, et al; American Academy of Child and Adolescent Psychiatry (AACAP) Committee on Quality Issues (CQI): Practice parameter for cultural competence in child and adolescent psychiatric practice. J Am Acad Child Adolesc Psychiatry 52(10):1101–1115, 2013 24074479

Rothe EM, Tzuang D, Pumariega AJ: Acculturation, development, and adaptation. Child Adolesc Psychiatr Clin N Am 19(4):681–696, 2010 21056341

Solomon A: Far from the Tree. New York, Scribner, 2013.

Think:Kids: The collaborative problem solving (CPS) approach. 2019. Available at: http://www.thinkkids.org/learn/our-collaborative-problem-solving-approach/. Accessed October 15, 2019.

Toppelberg CO, Collins BA: Language, culture, and adaptation in immigrant children. Child Adolesc Psychiatr Clin N Am 19(4):697–717, 2010 21056342

United Nations High Commission for Refugees: Global trends: forced displacement in 2017. 2017. Available at: http://www.unhcr.org/5b27be547.pdf. Accessed on October 15, 2019.

Volkan V: Immigrants and Refugees: Trauma, Perennial Mourning, Prejudice, and Border Psychology. New York, Routledge, 2018

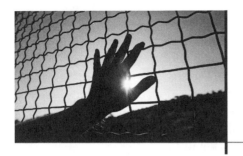

Chapter 8

ASYLUM SEEKERS

Mark Kinzie, M.D., Ph.D.

In 1967, the United Nations developed and approved the United Nations Protocol Relating to the Status of Refugees. The United States signed this treaty in 1968, and the U.S. Refugee Act was enacted by Congress in 1980. The Refugee Act was created to provide a systematic procedure for the admission of refugees into the United States and to provide comprehensive and uniform provisions for the effective resettlement of those refugees in the United States.

Under the Refugee Act, refugees are defined as any persons who have left the country in which they have citizenship or, if they are not a citizen of any country, have left their country of habitual residence and who are unable or unwilling to return to, and are unable or unwilling to avail themselves of the protection of, that country because of persecution or a well-founded fear of persecution on account of race, religion, nationality, membership in a particular social group, or political opinion. There is no universally agreed-on definition of persecution, but the harm does not have to be physical to constitute persecution. Harms ranging from economic to psychological to physical have been recognized by the courts as persecution (Meffert et al. 2016). Domestic violence has generally not been recognized as a qualifying harm.

There are two ways to be recognized as a refugee under the Refugee Act: either resettle to the United States as a refugee from abroad or present to the United States as an asylum seeker.

To resettle as a refugee, an individual must receive a referral from the U.S. Refugee Admissions Program. Applicants are interviewed by a U.S. Citizenship and Immigration Services (USCIS) officer to determine eligibility and are allowed to enter. Generally speaking, refugees entering the United States have official status and receive financial aid and medical support for 8 months.

Individuals fleeing persecution may arrive in the United States and apply for asylum as an asylum seeker. They attempt to enter the United States either with or without documentation allowing them to enter legally in order to make their claim. Asylum seekers receive no government support and may be deported if their asylum claim is denied. The asylum seeker may apply for work authorization after their case has been pending for 150 days. Although U.S. law provides arriving asylum seekers the right to be in the United States while their claim for protection is pending, in recent years the government has argued that it has the right to detain such individuals. Some courts have rejected this interpretation and have held that asylum seekers meeting certain criteria have a right to a hearing regarding their detention if they have been held for at least 6 months.

Once granted asylum, an asylee is protected from being returned to his or her home country, is authorized to work in the United States, and may apply for social benefits. An asylee may petition to bring his or her spouse and children to the United States. After 1 year, an asylee may apply for lawful permanent resident status.

Asylum is, therefore, a government-sanctioned protection granted to foreign nationals already in the United States or at the border who meet the legal definition of a refugee. As a signatory of the United Nations 1951 Convention Relating to the Status of Refugees and the 1967 Protocol and through U.S. law, the United States has legal obligations to provide protection to those who qualify as refugees.

SEEKING ASYLUM IN THE UNITED STATES

There are two primary ways in which a person may apply for asylum in the United States: by either applying affirmatively or defensively. An individual generally must apply for asylum within 1 year of arrival in the United States.

Affirmative applications are for a person who is not in removal proceedings. That is, it is the process for an individual who is lawfully present in the United States (on visa, for instance) or, if not lawfully present, who has not been apprehended by immigration authorities. An application for asylum is made through the USCIS, a division of the Department of Homeland Security (DHS). The applicant is interviewed by a USCIS asylum officer, who then makes a determination of eligibility. The interactions with the officer are meant to be "non-adversarial," meaning there is no attorney present representing the U.S. government. To the applicant, they can feel accusatory and often trigger memories of the persecution the applicant has fled in his or her country of origin. A supervisory asylum officer reviews the asylum officer's decision to ensure it is consistent with the law. Depending on the case, the supervisory asylum officer may refer the decision to asylum division staff at USCIS headquarters for additional review.

If the USCIS asylum officer does not grant the asylum application and the applicant does not have a lawful immigration status, the applicant is then referred to the immigration court for removal proceedings, where he or she may renew the request for asylum through the defensive process and appear before an immigration judge.

The defensive asylum process is for a person in removal proceedings. The defensive asylum seeker applies through the Executive Office for Immigration Review (EOIR), which is the office of the U.S. Department of Justice that is responsible for adjudicating all immigration cases in the United States. The EOIR oversees immigration courts in the United States through the Office of the Chief Immigration Judge. Immigration judges are thus employees of the Justice Department in the executive branch, rather than part of the judicial branch defined by Article 3 of the United States Constitution.

In the defensive asylum process, the asylum is sought as a "defense against removal" from the United States. The proceedings in immigration courts are adversarial—the judge hears not only the applicant's claim but also the arguments against eligibility by the U.S. Government represented by an Immigration and Customs Enforcement attorney. Asylum seekers do not necessarily have an attorney because they are not entitled to free representation (this being a court operated by the executive branch rather than judicial). All asylum seekers have the burden of proving that they meet the definition of a refugee. It is within these proceedings that mental health professionals are often asked to provide support for asylum seekers.

AFFIRMATIVE ASYLUM APPLICATION STATISTICS

As of March 2018, there were more than 318,000 affirmative asylum applications pending with USCIS and more than 690,000 open deportation cases. On average, these cases had been pending for 718 days and remained unresolved. Individuals with an immigration court case who were ultimately granted relief—such as asylum—by March 2018 waited more than 1,000 days on average for that outcome. New Jersey and California had the longest wait times, averaging 1,300 days until relief was granted in the immigration case. This author has seen cases of asylum seekers waiting longer than 10 years for their cases to be heard. In one case, because of a judge's illness, a case was postponed 18 months.

ROLE OF THE MENTAL HEALTH PROFESSIONAL

There are at least three ways in which a treating mental health professional can give assistance to patients applying for asylum: providing documentation of the effects of trauma, providing treatment of those effects, and providing testimony in immigration court.

In most cases, the psychiatrist should not be a patient's treating clinician and also act as an expert witness in court settings pertaining to the patient. The nature of the court, because it is under the executive branch of government, makes the proceedings less structured. The cost of hiring an additional examining expert witness is usually prohibitive to the asylum seeker, as well. In my experience, judges have permitted the treating clinician's testimony. In fact, judges have appreciated the long-term nature (typically years) of the clinical relationship and realize that a short examination is often insufficient.

DOCUMENTATION: GETTING A STORY

Getting the asylum seeker's story typically requires the development of a trusting relationship between the clinician and the asylum seeker. Because of the nature of the traumatic experience and posttraumatic stress disorder, patients are often reluctant to talk about the trauma. Discussing the trauma can exacerbate symptoms. Patients can be fearful that discussing their trauma could harm loved ones who remain in the environment in which the trauma has occurred. Patients may be unsure how the trauma story will be used and may fear that it will prevent them from getting asylum or government benefits. The process of asylum seeking and the use of the trauma story need to be explained to the patient.

Typically, interpreters are used during the interview. Interviewing of refugees requires competent and empathetic interpreters who can provide cultural information as well as interpretation of the language. Their role must be explained to the patient, and the patient must be assured that they are bound by the same rules of confidentiality as the clinician. In smaller, marginalized communities, interpreters may be known by the patient. The patient may know the interpreter's family or social status, preventing honest and open discussion of the case. These factors need to be explicitly discussed in order to create a safe and confidential environment for the patient.

Initial interviewing requires a slow and gentle approach. Patients are often intimidated by doctors and ashamed or traumatized about past behaviors or actions that they feel may be seen as reflecting poorly on them. Learning about patients from other cultures and appreciating them also helps reestablish the relationship. Clinicians should not retreat to "professional objectivity." This approach is usually seen by the patient as overly harsh and judgmental.

It is important to know about the patient's life before the trauma. The patient's socioeconomic status, education, and family support, as well as expectations about the trauma, all play an important role in the patient's response to the trauma and its psychological effects.

The role of the trauma story for treatment may be very different than the role of the story for the asylum case. Details regarding who perpetrated the trauma, when it occurred, and what the sequence of events was are more important in asylum cases. Knowing the patient's feelings of helplessness, expectations of rescue, and degree of family and societal support after the trauma is much more important in evaluation and treatment. The clinician's first aim is to support the mental health of the patient. Forensic details of the events can be clarified once the patient has been stabilized.

DIAGNOSIS

Because most asylum seekers have been traumatized and are fleeing additional trauma, PTSD is the most common diagnosis. Although documentation of the trauma story is of the utmost importance in court cases, for diagnosis and treatment, focusing on symptoms can be less intrusive to the patient and help stabilize him or her to be able to give more of the history. It is often easiest to ask first about lack of sleep and presence of nightmares. These symptoms can be addressed with medication, and this process can instill a sense of trust on the part of the patient that the clinician is concerned about the patient's well-being.

When a patient does report a history of trauma, it is important to document how that trauma correlates with mental health symptoms. Events that may be traumatizing to some people are not to others. Patients frequently report multiple traumatic events; some or all may leave lasting psychological symptoms. The correlation of trauma to symptoms is important in documenting the asylum case.

Severe PTSD is a chronic disorder with remissions and exacerbations. Patients often find relief during times of lower stress. Likewise, the symptoms may return with increased stress or events that serve as trauma reminders. Asylum seekers with PTSD frequently become more symptomatic before a court hearing not because of feigned symptoms, but rather because of the increased stress, the formality of the events reminding them of interactions with authority figures in their own country, and the fact that they will have to recite their trauma in a public setting.

Even in the presence of trauma, it is important not to neglect other diagnoses, especially major depressive disorder. The loss of family and supports in immigrating to a new culture can lead to demoralization and depression. The potentially lengthy time it takes to actually be granted asylum leads to hopelessness that their case will never be resolved and that they will never see their family again. Psychotic disorders from trauma can be seen as well. The intrusive memories and flashbacks can appear as auditory and visual hallucinations.

When a diagnosis is being made, it is important to focus on symptoms and the mental status examination. In addition to focusing on perceptual abnormalities, it is important to evaluate cognitive function. Traumatic brain injury in this population is common (Keatley et al. 2013).

Attorneys will often ask for the basis of the clinician's diagnosis. In most cases, the diagnosis will be determined exclusively by multiple clinical interviews over time. One reason for this approach is cost. Instruments and tests are expensive to use and interpret. However, the biggest reason concerns cultural validation. Most psychological batteries have not been validated for that patient's cultural, educational, economic, and medical background. The presence of a history of head trauma may also complicate interpretation of results.

A physical examination can be an important part of correlating a patient's reported history to its effects. Although many traumatic events are purely psychological in nature, physical trauma may create signature scars and deformities that can themselves act as triggers for traumatic memories. This clinician cared for a Somali patient who was thrown into a vat of boiling oil. The scars on her neck and hands served as frequent triggers of the traumatic event.

The Istanbul Protocol provides formal standards on assessing individuals who allege torture and ill treatment, investigating cases of alleged torture, and reporting the findings of such investigations to the judiciary and other bodies (Iacopino et al. 1999).

TREATMENT

As implied earlier in this chapter, treating symptoms early can help the patient gain trust in the clinician. The patient should be asked about which symptoms are most bothersome to him or her and let those be the initial focus of treatment.

Medicine can provide excellent relief of symptoms (see Chapter 5). Clonidine and prazosin can be used to address sleep and nightmares. Antidepressants can be used for depressive, anxiety, and PTSD symptoms. It is important to be clear with the patient about what medicine can and cannot do. Medications cannot erase the memories. They cannot make the actual circumstances of asylum seeking change. However, medications can reduce symptoms. Often when symptoms improve, difficulties that seemed insurmountable become manageable and solutions that seemed impossible become possible because of improved optimism.

Psychotherapy with asylum seekers can be very useful and important. A focus on grief and loss is often very helpful. A focus on the trauma with emphasis that the trauma is over and that triggered memories are not a recurrence of the trauma can be helpful as well. Supportive psychotherapy, with the goals of building new relationships, learning the new culture, and finding social supports, can help the patient with integration into the community.

TESTIMONY

Clinicians can help patients prepare to testify in immigration court. They can also provide supporting testimony on their patients' behalf.

Helping the Patient Prepare to Testify

The clinician can emphasize that providing testimony in court is difficult and that the patient's symptoms will naturally become worse given the stress and the stakes, but that the patient's symptoms will diminish once the testimony has been given and court is over. The clinician can also help attorneys by providing an explanation of the process and the clinician's role in it.

The clinician can also explain to the patient the expectations placed on the patient himself or herself. For instance, in many African cultures, looking down at the floor instead of at the judge is a sign of respect. To Americans, this appears to be an evasive sign of guilt.

Providing Testimony

In this author's experience, immigration courts are uniquely disarming environments where the proceedings have a much less formal feel than typical court proceedings. In some instances, more questions come from the judge than from the government lawyer. The tone is often conversational. It can be easy to forget that the stakes are high for the patient. It is important to remember that, despite appearances, conversations in the courtroom are on the record.

Some common questions asked of mental health professionals in immigration court are shown below. I have provided a few of the more common answers.

"Why did the asylum seeker wait beyond a year to apply for asylum or disclose her trauma history?"   By U.S. law, all individuals who apply for asylum must prove that they applied within 1 year of their arrival date into the United States. According to U.S. regulations, the 1-year deadline may be waived on the basis of changed or extraordinary circumstances. In some cases, patients simply are too fearful of thinking about the trauma. The trauma is too horrific and every time patients do anything related to that trauma (e.g., recounting the events, applying for asylum), they become increasing symptomatic. Therefore, denial of the event becomes the main way of coping. Avoidance of the trauma is a main symptom cluster of the PTSD. Other times, patients do not have a trusting relationship with the very people who could help. The attorney or the mental health clinician has not been able to create a safe environment for recounting the trauma. Patients may fear that telling the story may put loved ones at risk. They may also have had bad advice and simply did not know that they needed to disclose the trauma or were told that recounting the story would result in personal harm or put others at risk.

"Why does the asylum seeker appear evasive?"   Patients may appear evasive in their testimony because every time they try to talk about the trauma, their symptoms are readily triggered and they are trying to minimize them through avoidance or denial tactic. Patients may not know the complete story because of lapses in attention or consciousness during the initial traumatic event. As noted earlier, they may look evasive because of cultural expectations of respect (looking down or away at authority figures).

"Why is the story inconsistent with established facts?"   Sometimes, patients give incomplete histories of the events, get the sequence of events incorrect, or have verifiable errors in their histories. These inconsistencies and errors are actually normal and expected. Survivors of traumatic events often have difficulty remembering traumatic events. In an experiment conducted on soldiers trained in survival techniques who then went through interrogation (Morgan et al. 2004, 2013), the soldiers could not identify their interrogator in a line-up. This was in a controlled setting. In real-life traumatic experiences, the memory would even be worse.

"Why does the story change?" Memories are not set in stone; they are reconstructed and reinterpreted every time. Some facts can become confused. The sequence of events may be altered. This does not mean that the traumatic event did not happen.

"Is the asylum seeker malingering or lying?" Obviously, the clinician was not at the traumatic event. However, when a professional sees patients seeking asylum, particularly from the same country, the presentation can be consistent with others who have had similar experiences. The symptoms can be consistent with mental problems related to traumatic events. It is also very difficult to feign symptoms, diagnoses, and traumatic histories over the many years that it takes to become an asylum seeker.

TORTURE VICTIMS

Many asylum seekers have fled their country and have sought refuge because of torture. Because of this, it is necessary to understand what torture is and its consequences.

DEFINITIONS OF TORTURE

Torture is defined politically and legally rather than clinically. As such, whether a patient's trauma meets the criteria for torture is of great importance in immigration hearings. In terms of treatment of the patient, trauma and consequences are far more personal and subjective.

Torture is defined by the United Nations as:

> any act by which pain or suffering, whether physical or mental, is intentionally inflicted on a person for such purposes as obtaining from him or a third person information or a confession, punishing him for the act he or a third person has committed or is suspected of having committed, or intimidating or coercing him or a third person, or for any reason based on discrimination of any kind, when such pain or suffering is inflicted by or at the instigation of or with the consent or acquiescence of a public official or the person acting in an official capacity. It does not include pain or suffering arising only from, inherent in or incidental to lawful sanctions. (United Nations 1987)

The UN definition appears to exclude violence perpetrated by unofficial rebels or terrorists who ignore national or international mandates, random violence during war, and punishment allowed by national laws. Who perpetrates the violence is therefore a defining feature of the UN definition of torture.

The World Medical Association has a much more inclusive definition of torture. It defines torture as

> the deliberate, systematic or wanton infliction of physical or mental suffering by one or more persons acting alone or on the orders of any authority, to force another person to yield information, to make a confession, or for any other reason. (World Medical Association 2016)

In clinical settings, practitioners refer to violent acts as *trauma*. Trauma can have both medical and psychiatric definitions. In psychological terms, trauma refers to painful emotional experiences or shocks that can produce lasting psychological effects. Trauma occurs in situations in which one feels afraid and alone. At its most severe, trauma occurs when the external dangers converge with one's worst fears. For instance, severe trauma can occur when a person's fear of his or her imminent death seems probable.

Many factors are involved in traumatic situations that cause lasting psychological effects (R.S. Pynoos, personal communication, November 2003). Obviously, a person's appraisal of the situation and its threat is important. But, an appraisal of the patient's own response and degree of psychological control (e.g., keeping a cool head or losing control) will also play a role. Expectations of self-efficacy and outside interventions are factors, as is the experience of physical helplessness. Finally, an admission of helplessness and powerlessness will also contribute to the emergence of traumatic reexperiencing and PTSD symptoms.

Case I:Aryan

Aryan was a lawyer in Iran who protested against the government to the point that he was imprisoned. He suffered horrific traumatic experiences in prison, including having audio recordings of his wife and daughter being tortured constantly replayed in his solitary confinement cell. He begged to be released from solitary. Guards said that they would on the condition that he do them a favor. He agreed. At night, they drove him to another part of the prison where a man was blindfolded and tied to a post. They gave Aryan a gun and demanded that he shoot the blindfolded man. He did. Aryan was later haunted by the fact that rather than acting on his conscience and killing himself, he elected to kill the other man. The thought of his self-betrayal was a recurring flashback and nightmare for years.

TYPES OF TORTURE

Torture can take many physical forms. The trauma can be blunt or penetrating. The effects of burns, shocks, and extreme physical conditions such as forced body positions are all seen clinically. Sexual torture, including rape, is a common form. Mental torture can involve death threats, mock executions, solitary confinement, and sensory deprivation, including sleep deprivation.

CONSEQUENCES

For the Individual

Torture can cause virtually all psychiatric syndromes, including PTSD, social phobia, panic disorder, and other anxiety disorders. Psychotic disorders and dissociative states are also seen as a result of torture. In times of increased stress, unbearable reexperiencing of the torture can be triggered, leading to exacerbation of symptoms. In response to the symptoms, patients will attempt to cope by retreating and becoming isolated. Depression, substance use, and deliberate self-harm are attempts to soothe symptoms.

For Families

The usefulness of torture for governments and terrorist groups is that its effects extend beyond the individual being tortured. It can be a way to terrorize and control entire groups. As such, torture has familial and even transgenerational repercussions. The Bahá'ís of Iran are a group who have suffered at the hands of torture. There are roughly 300,000 Bahá'ís of Iran, and their leaders have been tortured and executed because of their faith and their perceived threat to the Iranian government.

Case 2: Mansoor

Mansoor was a Bahá'í of Iran patient seen by the author. He was 45 years old and had been married to Zanib for 20 years. They were cousins, and the marriage was arranged. In Iran, Mansoor had a successful construction business. After the Iranian Revolution, his father was imprisoned and the family's property was confiscated. Mansoor was jailed on multiple occasions, during which he was beaten and subjected to mock executions and witnessed the execution of others. He was a recent arrival to the United States and was sleeping 2–3 hours a night and had nightmares every night. He was anhedonic, with hypervigilance and an exaggerated startle response. He also was avoidant and depressed. His chief complaint was his lack of ability to show love and feelings toward his family, which led to withdrawing from others and eventual drug use.

Zanib, Mansoor's wife, was 37 years old. Before they married, life was very difficult. When she was 15 years old, a cousin was killed by government officials, but the family was blamed. She had been depressed for as long as she could remember and suffered from constant fatigue and irritability. She also had nonepileptic seizure events.

Ashkan, 20 years old, was the couple's oldest son. When he was 10 years old, he saw his mother having a seizure and thought she was dying. He never recovered from it and lived in constant fear of his mother's death. He felt that he had no parents and could trust no one. Ashkan himself suffered from depression and panic attacks. His chief complaint was anger at his father and feeling lost.

FEMALE GENITAL MUTILATION

Female genital mutilation, also called "female circumcision," affects about 130 million women worldwide. It occurs mostly in Africa, the Middle East, and Southwest Asia. It has been estimated that the prevalence in Somalia is about 98%.

TYPES OF FEMALE GENITAL MUTILATION

The World Health Organization (2008) has defined female genital mutilation as comprising procedures that involve partial or total removal of the external female genitalia for nonmedical reasons. The WHO has classified female genital mutilation into four types:

- Type I: excision of the prepuce with or without excision of part or all of the clitoris ("Sunna circumcision")
- Type II: excision of the clitoris together with partial or total excision of the labia minora
- Type III: excision of part or all of the external genitalia and stitching/narrowing of the vaginal opening (infibulation)
- Type IV: all other harmful procedures to the female genitalia for nonmedical purposes

Infibulation is the most common form of female genital mutilation in Somalia.

PSYCHOLOGICAL EFFECTS

Two studies suggest that rates of PTSD and anxiety disorders are higher in women who have undergone female genital mutilation. A 2005 study by Behrendt and Moritz looked at 23 circumcised Senegalese women in Dakar. The authors found a higher prevalence of PTSD and other psychiatric disorders compared with the circumcised women. Knipscheer et al. (2015) found that a third of the 66 immigrant African women with female genital mutilation had symptoms that met criteria for affective and anxiety disorders, including PTSD.

Attitudes regarding female genital mutilation have changed with time in non–female genital mutilation–performing countries. A study of Somali men and women in London found that living in Britain from a younger age was associated with abandonment of female genital mutilation (Morison et al. 2004).

In this author's experience, older Somali women in the United States will say that female genital mutilation was the right choice for them. It was expected and there was a great deal of support from the family and community for it. However, they would not endorse their granddaughters having it performed.

Case 3: Meelaaney

Meelaaney was a 20-year-old Somali woman who had been in the United States for about 5 years. She presented with depression and panic attacks. Her chief complaint was depression, irritability, and identity problems in the setting of conflicts with her family. Her family was unhappy that she was dating an American man and that she was not respecting Somali traditions. She was born in Somalia and lived in a refugee camp in Kenya. As a teenager, she immigrated to Germany without her family and was there for 2 years. She was very bright and acculturated rapidly. She learned German quickly and even joined a German dance team. When she was 12, she underwent infibulation. She was very calm throughout the procedure, but her sister was not. Her sister aggressively refused the procedure and ended up not having it. After the female genital mutilation, Meelaaney had high degrees of anxiety and panic and became distant from her family and culture. However, at her mother's insistence, she immigrated to the United States to rejoin her family. Her symptoms of anxiety and depression became worse after she started dating the American man and her memories and anger regarding the female genital mutilation resurfaced. Treatment terminated after she moved in with her boyfriend and limited her contact with family. Her symptoms improved.

KEY CLINICAL POINTS

- Individuals who are fleeing persecution may arrive in the United States and apply for asylum as asylum seekers. Asylum seekers receive no government support and may be deported if their asylum claim is denied.

- Asylum seekers have the right to be in the United States while their claim is pending; however, some recent government attorneys have argued that the U.S. Government has the right to detain such individuals.

- The legal process involving asylum seekers, their acceptance or rejection, and potential deportation is complicated and lengthy. The process creates much stress for the asylees and usually exacerbates their symptoms.

- The psychiatrist can provide help for patients who are applying for asylum: by providing documentation of the effects of trauma, providing treatments for the effects, and providing testimony in immigration court.

- For asylum cases, details about trauma, such as when the trauma occurred and what events preceded it and in what sequence, are more germaine.

- Providing testimony, the psychiatrist faces common questions: "Why does the asylum seeker appear evasive?" "Why is the story inconsistent with established facts?" "Why does the story change?"

- A special case is a victim of torture, defined as "the deliberate, systematic, or wanton infliction of physical or mental suffering by one or more persons acting alone or on the orders of any authority, to force another person to yield information, to make a confession, or for any other reason." Victims of torture can usually make a case for successful asylum.

REFERENCES

Behrendt A, Moritz S: Posttraumatic stress disorder and memory problems after female genital mutilation. Am J Psychiatry 162(5):1000–1002, 2005 15863806

Iacopino V, Ozkalipçi O, Schlar C, et al: The Istanbul Protocol: international standards for the effective investigation and documentation of torture and ill treatment. Lancet 354(9184):1117, 1999 10509518

Keatley E, Ashman T, Im B, Rasmussen A: Self-reported head injury among refugee survivors of torture. J Head Trauma Rehabil 28(6):E8–E13, 2013 23348404

Knipscheer J, Vloeberghs E, van der Kwaak A, et al: Mental health problems associated with female genital mutilation. BJPsych Bull 39(6):273–277, 2015 26755984

Meffert SM, Shome S, Neylan TC, et al: Health impact of human rights testimony: harming the most vulnerable? BMJ Glob Health Jul 21;1(1):e000001, 2016 28588904

Morgan CA 3rd, Hazlett G, Doran A, et al: Accuracy of eyewitness memory for persons encountered during exposure to highly intense stress. Int J Law Psychiatry 27(3):265–279, 2004 15177994

Morgan CA 3rd, Southwick S, Steffian G, et al: Misinformation can influence memory for recently experienced, highly stressful events. Int J Law Psychiatry 36:11–17, 2013

Morison LA, Dirir A, Elmi S, et al: How experiences and attitudes relating to female circumcision vary according to age on arrival in Britain: a study among young Somalis in London. Ethn Health 9(1):75–100, 2004 15203466

Refugee Act of 1980. Pub L 96-212. 94 Stat 102. 17 March 1980

United Nations: Convention against Torture and Other Cruel, Inhuman or Degrading Treatment or Punishment. Adopted December 10, 1984. Effective June 26, 1987. Available at: https://www.ohchr.org/EN/ProfessionalInterest/Pages/CAT.aspx. Accessed October 28, 2019.

World Health Organization: Eliminating Female Genital Mutilation: An Interagency Statement—OHCHR, UNAIDS, UNDP, UNECA, UNESCO, UNFPA, UNHCR, UNICEF, UNIFEM, WHO. Geneva, World Health Organization, 2008

World Medical Association: WMA Declaration of Tokyo: Guidelines for Physicians Concerning Torture and Other Cruel, Inhuman or Degrading Treatment or Punishment in Relation to Detention and Imprisonment. Revised Version, October 2016. Available at: https://www.wma.net/policies-post/wma-declaration-of-tokyo-guidelines-for-physicians-concerning-torture-and-other-cruel-inhuman-or-degrading-treatment-or-punishment-in-relation-to-detention-and-imprisonment. Accessed October 28, 2019.

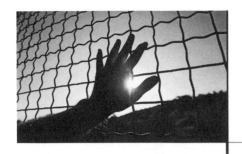

Chapter 9

GERIATRIC PSYCHIATRIC PROBLEMS AMONG REFUGEES

Paul Leung, M.D.
J. David Kinzie, M.D., FACPsych, DLFAPA

With a worldwide aging population, there is increasing concern about the physical and mental problems facing the geriatric population. Little has been written about the geriatric refugee population, but there is growing agreement that older refugees face worse outcomes and greater difficulty accessing medical services and treatment. Among older Kurdish refugees in the United States, 67% had depression (Cummings et al. 2011). Their depression was associated with the stresses of migratory grief, death of a spouse, medical disability, lower income, lower English proficiency, and the aging process. Holocaust survivors in Australia were

The authors appreciate the help from Kim Truong-Pham, M.S., and Loan Huynh, L.C.S.W., with preparation of this chapter.

119

found to have increased anxiety, worsening of PTSD symptoms, cognitive declines, and increased cardiometabolic diseases as they aged (Paratz and Katz 2011).

In this chapter we explore the issues facing geriatric refugees with dementia, especially among the Vietnamese refugee population. Many older ethnic-minority adults face culturally associated barriers that make it more difficult for them to receive a diagnosis of dementia. Additionally, they have more severe cognitive and behavioral impairments when they present for their initial evaluation compared with their non-Hispanic white counterparts (Sayegh and Knight 2013). Vietnamese in Australia face greater hurdles in accessing dementia services, and this was found to be associated with greater caregiver burden, higher rates of mortality and morbidity, and increased rates of hospitalization (Xiao et al. 2015). By explaining these difficulties, we seek to emphasize the need for culturally and linguistically appropriate dementia services as well as the importance of educating patients' families and caregivers in a culturally sensitive manner.

INTERCULTURAL PSYCHIATRIC PROGRAM

The Intercultural Psychiatric Program, or IPP, began over 40 years ago initially to treat the refugee Vietnamese population fleeing wartime and postwar Vietnam. Many of these initial patients from the 1970s and 1980s are still being treated at IPP to this day. Although increasingly the patients treated at the clinic are from Africa and the Middle East, Vietnamese refugees are still the largest group in the patient population, with 239 patients, or almost 25% of the clinic's total patient population. Of these 239 patients, 86 are at least 65 years or older. Among this group of patients, medical and psychiatric conditions are widespread and severe. A random survey of 25 Vietnamese patients 65 years or older yielded the diagnoses shown in Table 9–1.

Six patients, or nearly a quarter of the sample group, have dementia. It should be noted that many geriatric Vietnamese in general may already have dementia but have not had a diagnosis or sought treatment for it. In our clinical experience, patients with PTSD have a higher prevalence of dementia, which is a finding supported by others as well (Mohlenhoff et al. 2017). The number of our patients with schizophrenia is surprisingly high for a refugee clinic; however, it should be noted that many of our patients started treatment at our clinic when they were much younger specifically for their schizophrenia, in some cases over 40 years ago.

TABLE 9–1. Diagnoses of Intercultural Psychiatric Program Vietnamese geriatric patient population, ages 65–90 years (*N*=25)

Diagnosis	*n*
Psychiatric	
PTSD and depression	8
PTSD alone	1
Depression alone	7
Schizophrenia	9
Dementia	6
Medical	
Hypertension	5
Diabetes	2
Diabetes and hypertension	2

MANAGEMENT

When an elderly patient presents with dementia, the first priority is to determine if the dementia is the result of other health issues and then, if possible, to treat those issues. Although dementia itself cannot be cured, treating its underlying medical causes can lessen its progression or even prevent it from getting worse. Therefore, it is important to conduct a thorough medical evaluation as well as a psychiatric and social history of the patient when he or she initially seeks treatment. For example, many elderly refugee patients suffer from hypertension and diabetes and take multiple medications to treat their condition and/or symptoms. Patients and their families are often unaware of the purpose of prescribed medications. Many medicines, both psychiatric and medical, have anticholinergic side effects and can cause confusion or additional memory problems. Health care providers should ask about all medicines the patient is taking, but it is even more effective to have the patient or his or her family members bring in the medicine to be physically inspected.

Once the patient is medically stabilized, the next step is to manage the patient's symptoms of dementia and maintain his or her quality of life. The brunt of this effort will most likely be taken on by the patient's family members. As such, it is important to educate the family members and give them guidance and support. They need to understand that dementia has no cure but that effective treatments exist for the symptoms of dementia. These treatments can minimize disruption to their and the patient's life, thereby alleviating stress on the family members and helping the patient feel more comfortable.

It is useful to ask the family what they see as the patient's most disruptive behaviors or symptoms. A very common complaint is the patient yelling at night or wandering around. Psychosis with irritability is another common complaint. Barring a separate medical cause for these symptoms, a medication such as trazodone is useful as a sleep aid. If PTSD is still present in the patient, it is important to continue treatment with a selective serotonin reuptake inhibitor (SSRI), clonidine, or prazosin, because these can help with nightmares and aid in sleep (Boehnlein and Kinzie 2007).

A counselor who is linguistically and culturally competent in the patient's cultural and ethnic background is essential to providing treatment. Not only can counselors assist in translating, they can, with their cultural knowledge, help healthcare providers navigate issues that arise from cultural beliefs and social practices. For example, in our experience many Vietnamese refugee patients and their families believe that dementia is a result of their refugee experience and thus blame themselves for their condition. It is useful for these patients and their families to know that dementia, as well as other mental health problems, is quite common in mainstream society and is not their fault.

Another issue that providers may encounter is significant resistance or reluctance to follow the provider's advice for treatment. This often stems from traditions or beliefs that make the patients and their families see illness as shameful or dishonorable. One example is the reluctance among Asian families to place a relative in a nursing home, which we will discuss in further detail later in this chapter. With a culturally competent counselor on hand, health care providers can address these concerns or even preempt such problems with education and better communication.

Guiding principles in caring for patients with dementia include having as few restrictions on their activities as possible and encouraging socialization and group activities. There is a natural tendency for families of dementia patients to restrict the patient's movements in order to better control him or her. Such restriction can have severe negative consequences on the patient's quality of life and should be discouraged. However, family members must also be educated to know when to be more restrictive, such as when the dementia patient wanders away too often.

Socialization and group activities have multiple benefits, both for the patient and for the family caretakers. For the patient, it prevents social isolation and establishes healthy structure in his or her life. Here at the IPP clinic, we encourage socialization activities during group therapy, and have noted that our patients feel a sense of belonging and participate in a safe social network, even with our most impaired patients. Activities such as group lessons about American life can also help elderly refugees establish and maintain social skills. There are noteworthy examples of this in our clinic's weekly Vietnamese socialization groups. With such activities, patients may even functionally improve. Such activities also benefit family members, because it gives them regular time off, helping to alleviate caregiver stress and burnout.

Case 1: A Widowed Vietnamese Woman

An 87-year-old widowed Vietnamese woman was referred to the IPP clinic after an admission to an inpatient ward at a nearby hospital. She was admitted for hallucinations, talking to herself, religious preoccupation, and chasing "the devil in her house" with a knife. During her admission she responded to perphenazine, and she regularly visited our clinic for treatment up until 1996. She did not return to our clinic until 2005 but has continued receiving treatment at our clinic ever since. The woman's return was prompted by her family's concern about her confusion and agitation that had caused one of her daughters to quit work in order to take care of the patient. It is of note that she also had two sons, both of whom have a history of schizophrenia. What exactly caused the family's concern is not clear. When the patient returned, she continued with perphenazine at a low dose of 8 mg, but she had no hallucinations or pressured speech, nor did she have any ideas of reference.

In 2012, at the age of 81, the patient, according to her records, had poor memory and poor concentration; however, she had no psychotic symptoms. In time her memory continued to worsen, and she frequently needed to be reminded where she was or what activity she was doing at the moment. She also became more paranoid, frequently accusing people of stealing her things. She continued to live with her children. By 2018, at age 87, she no longer recognized her grandchildren. The family continues to be able to take care of her as long as she receives psychiatric treatment and her major symptoms are under control. However, the patient's memory and concentration impairments have severely affected her and her family's lives.

This patient has a long-term history of schizophrenia that has been mostly under control through treatment, subsequently combined with a later onset of dementia. Her new psychotic symptoms of hallucinations and delusions developed as a result of her dementia.

TRAUMA OF FORMER MEMBERS OF SOUTH VIETNAM GOVERNMENT FORCES

Within the Vietnamese refugee population, there is a subset who served in South Vietnam's armed forces and law enforcement who were held in "re-education" camps after the Communist North Vietnamese government took control of the country. These camps were a brutal experience for internees. Victims suffered beatings, starvation, diseases, and forced labor and were imprisoned between 3 and 9 years. In many camps the mortality rate was greater than 50%. Those able to return home and reunite with their families came back wounded, emaciated, and psychologically traumatized by their experience. However, returning home gave them little relief because their status as former enemies of the new government meant that they and their families would face continued persecution from the government. Families of former soldiers were stripped of their property, forced to move to inhospitable areas to fend for themselves, denied access to basic services such as health care and education, and prevented from obtaining employment to support themselves. In such an environment, there was little chance for these former internees to receive help for their psychological and medical traumas.

At the IPP clinic, we have treated 15 geriatric patients who went through the re-education camps. They range in age from 64 to 84 years. Thirteen out of the 15 still have ongoing PTSD and receive treatment for ongoing nightmares. Seven have neurocognitive disorders or dementia. Eleven have hypertension and 8 have diabetes. The survivors of these camps suffer from severe medical and psychological problems, as have other survivors of concentration camps, such as during the Holocaust.

Case 2: An Older, Married Vietnamese Man

The patient, a 71-year-old Vietnamese man, has been coming to the IPP clinic since 1983. Originally, he was referred to our clinic for evaluation after being hospitalized for depression with some suicidal thoughts. During the evaluation, he reported that he also experienced nightmares, had very poor sleep, and would frequently wake up at night. He also had flashbacks about the war in Vietnam about twice a day, felt paranoid when people were near him, and imagined explosions going off around him. It was clear that the patient had PTSD, and an examination of his personal history revealed that he was a former police officer in South Vietnam during the war. After the war ended, he was detained in a re-education camp between 1975 and 1980. He was beaten constantly by the camp guards, suffered harsh and deprived conditions, and lost a great deal of weight because of starvation. He also witnessed countless detainees dying in the camps. After he was released from the camp and reunited with his family, the government forcibly relocated them to "new economic zones," essentially remote pieces of land deep in the wilderness where the families were left to fend for themselves.

In treatment at our clinic, the patient presented with multiple medical problems, including tachycardia arrhythmia and gout. In 2005, he was diagnosed with diabetes and hypertension. Treatment included SSRIs and, on occasion, the use of antipsychotic medications. In general, his psychiatric symptoms remained stable despite having multiple medical issues. In 2014, at the age of 67, the patient reported having problems with memory, Subsequent cognitive testing showed impairment of his short-term memory. His memory worsened as time went on to the point that he could not drive unless someone was with him to help him navigate. Even as his memory became more and more impaired, he continued to come to the clinic for individual therapy and to participate in group sessions, although he remained socially isolated. In his 25 years of treatment the patient's PTSD symptoms have been reduced through medications.

However, his increasing age has led to new medical problems such as his neurocognitive impairment. The patient's afflictions and poor health are the result of ongoing trauma stemming from his experience during and after the war in Vietnam as well as the difficulty of adjusting to life in the United States (Kinzie et al. 2008). Other members of South Vietnamese government forces will have similar medical issues because they have similar traumatic histories.

THE FAMILY IN AGONY

In many Asian cultures, there is a long-held tradition of all family members taking care of the family elders. Traditionally, the entire family would work together to care for older members, each chipping in time and effort to make sure the elders are well-cared for at home. For many refugees from these cultures, settling in America has dramatically disrupted this traditional practice. Many refugee families experience financial difficulties that require all members of the family to work in order to make ends meet, constraining how much time they can collectively spend on caretaking. Finding work may also require family members to spread out across the country, reducing the number of people who can come to help when needed. Compared with life in the home country, it is much less likely that extended family members will be able to help an elderly relative. When an elderly patient suffers from a condition that requires constant long-term care, such as a terminal illness or dementia, the burden is borne by the immediate family members. This dramatically increases the family members' workload, stress, and feelings of helplessness and anxiety.

Health care providers often recommend to families that they place their elderly relative in a nursing home that can provide better monitoring and care. However, traditional Asian cultural values consider this as essentially abandoning the relative, which would bring shame and criticism on the rest of the family. As a result, families will be reluctant or unwilling to follow this advice. Proper education and the ability to place the elderly person in a culturally and linguistically appropriate setting will greatly ease the family's concerns and increase their willingness to place their relative in a long-term-care facility.

Case 3: The 86-Year-Old Grandmother

The patient had suffered a stroke about 1 year previously and still had weakness on the left side of her body, but she was able to walk slowly with a walker. Because she was at risk of falling and injuring herself, she needed to be monitored throughout the day. Her memory deteriorated in comparison to her baseline status the previous year. There were times she walked out of the house and could not find her way home. She would turn on the stove but then walk away, leaving it unattended. She slept mostly during the day and stayed awake during the night. She constantly accused others of stealing from her because she could not remember where she had left her belongings. She became increasingly confused and frequently had fits of anger. She made threats against people at home because she believed they wanted her dead.

The patient's doctor recognized that her dementia had reached an advanced stage and suggested to the patient's family that she be placed in a memory care facility. The family initially expressed great resistance to this advice, arguing that they could not abandon their grandmother. They feared that she would be neglected and maybe even die in the care of such a facility because she lacked the ability to speak in English and would be unable to communicate with the staff. A social worker from IPP who spoke the same language and came from the same cultural background as the patient met with family members to address their concerns. After multiple meetings, the social worker was able to explain to the family how important it was to have professional care on a continuous basis to ensure the patient's safety. The social worker also encouraged the family to make a plan for family members to visit the grandmother daily in rotation to ensure that she was properly cared for at the facility. Eventually, the family found a nursing home facility that had Asian language staff and could provide Asian meals for their clients. With their fears assuaged, the family agreed to place their grandmother in the facility.

CONCLUSION

As refugee populations age, geriatric issues inevitably will arise among them. Addressing these issues, especially dementia, and providing treatment will be a difficult and complicated challenge for health care providers, patients, and their families. Much of this burden will be taken on by the patient's family. Because of this, the primary goal of treatment is to educate the family about dementia and its related problems. This knowledge will help families care for patients at home and improve patients' quality of life. Psychoeducation can also help families feel less anxious when they encounter disturbing behavior or severe memory problems. When given appropriate skills, families can manage disruptive behavior, enabling patients to stay at home and lessening stress on family members.

To this end, it is essential that a counselor with the necessary cultural and language skills be present when the clinician is evaluating the patient and educating the family members. These counselors act as the bridge between the patient's family and the medical team, not only to translate but also to provide context and navigate cultural issues and nuances. Culturally competent counselors help patients and their families feel assured that their concerns are understood and help providers to ensure that treatment is properly followed.

Patients should also be given opportunities to socialize and participate in group activities. This will prevent them from becoming isolated, and it will give them social support and provide structure to their life. Such activities can help improve symptoms and maintain a high quality of life for both patients and their families. These benefits are even more robust when social activities and groups are in the same cultural and language group as the patient's. A culturally and linguistically competent counselor can help patients' families and providers find such activities.

KEY CLINICAL POINTS

- As the refugee population ages, many refugees will have aging-related problems, especially dementia.

- Because of cultural barriers, many families will have difficulties accessing services for their aging parents.
- Severe trauma, along with the resultant PTSD, probably increases the prevalence of dementia among elderly refugees.
- In the experience of Vietnamese, and increasingly other, refugee groups, all or most families want to keep their elderly, no matter how severe the dementia, at home.
- Educating the family and supporting the caregivers is the main treatment for elderly issues.
- Social groups with patients of the same ethnicity can decrease dislocation anxiety and give the family some relief.

■────────────────────────────────■

REFERENCES

Boehnlein JK, Kinzie JD: Pharmacologic reduction of CNS noradrenergic activity in PTSD: the case for clonidine and prazosin. J Psychiatr Practice 13(2):72–78, 2007 17414682

Cummings S, Sull L, Davis C, et al: Correlates of depression among older Kurdish. Soc Work 56(2):159–169, 2011 21553579

Kinzie JD, Riley C, McFarland B, et al: High prevalence rates of diabetes and hypertension among refugee psychiatric patients. J Nerv Ment Dis 196(2):108–112, 2008 21553579

Mohlenhoff BS, O'Donovan A, Weiner MW, et al: Dementia risk in posttraumatic stress disorder: the relevance of sleep-related abnormalities in brain structure, amyloid, and inflammation. Curr Psychiatry Rep 19(11):89, 2017 29035423

Paratz ED, Katz B: Ageing Holocaust survivors in Australia. Med J Aust 194(4):194–197, 2011 21401461

Sayegh P, Knight BG: Cross-cultural differences in dementia: the Sociocultural Health Belief Model. Int Psychogeriatr 25(4):517–530, 2013 23237243

Xiao LD, Habel L, De Bellis A: Perceived challenges in dementia care by Vietnamese family caregivers and care workers in South Australia. J Cross Cult Gerontol 30(3):333–352, 2015 25935206

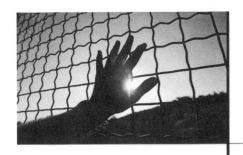

Chapter 10

CONTEMPORARY REFUGEE CRISIS AT THE UNITED STATES– MEXICO BORDER

Bernardo Ng, M.D., FAPA
Erike Apolinar, LMFT
Mario A. Martinez, M.D.

In this chapter we provide a recounting of a humanitarian crisis that developed in 2018 and remained unresolved by the time of the writing of this chapter. This crisis left asylum seekers migrating from Central America to the United States "stuck" in Mexico, more specifically in the city of Tijuana, right at the border between California (United States) and Baja California (Mexico). The crisis became known worldwide, with numerous news sources, academicians, politicians, and nongovernmental organizations highlighting the legal, geopolitical, trade, financial, moral, ethical, humanitarian, medical, and mental health issues implicated in this crisis. High numbers of these asylum seekers ended up "caught" between two countries, away from their home and yet unable to enter the country chosen as their final destination.

You will read a chronological description of the events, based on news media sources, as they became known to the general public. In order to illustrate the reality that many of these asylum seekers are running away from, we have included two clinical cases of female minors; one treated in the United States and the other one treated in Mexico. We begin the chapter by describing the features of the United States–Mexico border region.

THE UNITED STATES–MEXICO BORDER REGION

The border between the United States and Mexico is one of the longest in the world. Extending from the southern tip of the state of Texas to the coast of the state of California, the border is approximately 2,000 miles in length. The territory comprising 62.5 miles north and south of this boundary is recognized by the United States Department of Health and Human Services as the U.S.-Mexico border region (UMBR). The population in this region is estimated to be approximately 15 million, including people from 25 Native American Nations; the population is expected to double by the year 2025. It involves four states (California, Arizona, New Mexico, Texas) representing near 70 million people, including 154 Native American tribes, and 2 of the 10 fastest-growing metropolitan areas (Laredo and McAllen) in the United States. Additionally, there are six states (Baja California, Sonora, Chihuahua, Coahuila, Nuevo León, Tamaulipas), 80 municipalities, and almost 20 million people on the Mexican side. As dynamic as this region seems to be, the majority of the population can be described as having unfavorable health and social conditions and is medically underserved, with professional health shortages, higher rates of uninsured people, higher poverty, and higher migration rates than the median within their corresponding states.

The UMBR has 15 pairs of sister cities, such as Nuevo Laredo–Laredo, El Paso–Ciudad Juárez, and of course San Diego–Tijuana, where the events described in this chapter took place (U.S. Department of Health and Human Services 2017). Numerous attempts have been made to achieve binational regional cooperation to address public health demands, as the border can hardly control, prevent, or modify how culture, religion, occupation, and other social determinants influence numerous health conditions, such as diabetes, tuberculosis, substance use, and suicide (Carrillo et al. 2017; Hernandez-Fuentes et al. 2013). An unfortunate example is how, on any given day, heroin users on the American side go into the Mexican side to buy methamphetamine to "complement" their dose in the form of "speed balling" and return to the United States before sundown. As well, young people cross the border with "small" supplies of marihuana that is now legal in California, to share or sell with friends on the Mexican side (Ng et al. 2018).

But why Tijuana and not any other city in the UMBR? Tijuana was founded in 1920. Hollywood stars, actors, musicians, and producers were looking for a place where they could drink unaffected by the Volstead Act. The casinos, bars, and hotels that developed accordingly hired all kinds of workers. Almost 100 years later, with a population of 3 million, the city of Tijuana has evolved in its culture, entertainment, cuisine, industry, and education, and also in the number of homeless persons, uninsured, drug users, undocumented migrants, and deportees from the United States. As Roberto Castillo Udiarte described his experience, "En Tijuana todos somos migrantes, la única diferencia es que unos llegamos antes y otros llegamos después [In Tijuana we are all migrants; the only difference is that some of us arrived before and some of us arrived later]" (Castillo Udiarte et al. 2016).

THE "VIA CRUCIS" CARAVAN

During the 2016 presidential race, then–Republican candidate Donald Trump announced as one of his most important promises the building of a wall at the southern border to prevent undocumented immigrants from entering American soil. Soon after taking office, he signed an executive order to improve border security, and among other measures he insisted on was the construction of a wall to deter illegal immigration from Latin America and other regions of the world (The White House 2017). Toward the end of 2017 prototypes for such a wall were approved, to be built at a cost of $20 million dollars, in an attempt to have funding for the complete project approved (Guild 2017). The prototypes were built and eventually destroyed, before a budget was approved (Associated Press 2019). During the 2018 State of the Union address he presented the four pillars of his proposal on immigration reform: a path to citizenship for 1.8 million people already in the United States, the end of the visa lottery, the end of chain migration, and securing of the southern border with the construction of a wall (CNN 2018). Toward the end of 2018, President Trump insisted that Mexico had to do more to prevent migration into the United States, and it was expected that great progress was going to be achieved once then–President-Elect of Mexico

Andrés Manuel López Obrador took office. Shortly after, the "remain in Mexico" policy between Mexico and the United States became popular news. Reputable news media sources published numerous stories about how the governments of the two countries were going to reach or not reach an agreement around such a policy. Although no official agreement became public, the idea was that asylum seekers from the poorest countries in Central America and the Caribbean were to be "held" in Mexico for weeks to months or even longer as their applications were being processed prior to entering the United States. It also became public that if the Mexican government was unwilling to go along, the United States government would completely close the border (Partlow and Miroff 2018). Months later, toward the end of the spring of 2019 under the pressure of applying increasing tariffs on Mexican goods imported to the United States, the two countries reached a "deal" in which the government of Mexico agreed to increase the presence of federal law enforcement officials at the border with Guatemala, increase actions against human traffickers and criminal smugglers, deter illegal immigration, and expand the "remain in Mexico" policy so that asylum seekers would have to stay in Mexico until their applications for asylum in the United States were approved or denied. So, it finally happened that those seeking asylum in United States soil will have to use Mexico as the "waiting room" until their turn comes to have their application processed (CBS News 2019).

Along with President Trump's anti-immigrant plans and remarks, it would have been expected that the flow of immigrants would progressively decrease. It seemed to go that way during President Trump's first year in office, but after that, the number of apprehensions at the border increased. According to the U.S. Customs and Border Protection website, the number of total apprehensions of inadmissible entries in 2016 was 553,378. That number went down to 415,517 in 2017, which coincides with President Trump's campaign and first year in office, only to go back up in 2018 to 521,090, with an unprecedented rise of 676,315 by May 2019. During May 2019 alone, there were 144,278 apprehensions (U.S. Customs and Border Protection 2019).

During the second part of 2018, migrants from the Central America northern triangle—namely, Guatemala, Honduras, and El Salvador—organized to migrate in a caravan northward through Mexico into the United States. This caravan was named "Via Crucis" emulating Jesus Christ's walk on the day of his crucifixion. The movement became known worldwide, with an evident polarization of public opinion among citizens from Mexico and the United States. Either by foot, train, or bus the migrants made it to the city of Tijuana, Mexico, first by the hundreds and eventually the thousands. Although without actual disclosure of the sources of support, the media reported that these migrants, unlike other asylum seekers, were receiving support from immigration attorneys, nonprofit organizations, and even regular American citizens touched by the movement and the critical conditions in their home countries (Esténs 2018).

The city of Tijuana became the final destination within Mexico. Local city officials set up shelters for the migrants who crossed the entire country in the hope of entering the United States. During the first days after their arrival, numerous appearances in different parts of the existing wall became news. Tension increased among the citizens and residents of Tijuana overwhelmed with the nearly 7,000 migrants who had arrived in a matter of weeks only to find shelters that totaled less than 1,000 beds (La Jeunesse 2018).

Entire families of migrants were present on the south side of the border, guarded by Mexican federal police officers, while National Guard and U.S. Border Patrol officers stood on the northern side. All parties became both witnesses and protagonists in images that traveled around the world. Meanwhile, the overextended city of Tijuana, running out of resources for food and lodging, as well as clothing, education, health, and safety, did not disturb the celebratory mood of the caravanners, who felt so close to their dream becoming true.

In the heat of their arrival, migrants approached the existing 26-foot-tall dark brown wall between the two countries, made of approximately 10-inch-wide metal columns that are tightly welded to one another. These columns have about 4 inches of space between each other, allowing bystanders to see onto the other side. Some caravanners actually climbed the wall, others chanted, and others were just watching, as they could actually see "American soil" on the other side (Moore and Almond 2019). Their understanding was that they had all it takes to qualify as refugees; either well informed or not, they were expectant and hopeful. By the third day, while growing numbers of people gathered on the Mexican side, the world saw tensions rise and watched as the situation escalated with the shooting of several charges of tear gas, obligating the crowd to disperse in fear. Dozens of gas canisters were visible on the Mexican side of the border. The reports stated that officers responded to migrants throwing projectiles and/or rocks toward them and thus were acting within protocol (Specia and Gladstone 2018).

Nonetheless, academicians argued that international treaties such as the United Nations Charter regarding sovereign rights and obligations of members' countries state that members shall refrain in their international relations from the threat or use of force against the territorial integrity of other members. The shooting of tear gas was qualified as use of nonlethal yet disproportionate force. Beyond the academic and intellectual discourse, this use of force also became a moral and humanitarian issue. Although public opinion might have been polarized in both countries regarding illegal migration and asylum seeking, the most common response was one of disapproval, both by large organizations and by individuals, with statements such as "there were children around, and some of them even in diapers" (Specia and Gladstone 2018).

It has been argued that most of the members of this caravan did not only come from economically deprived environments but were also escaping from dangerous and crime ridden communities (Altman et al. 2018; Keller et al. 2017). The following cases illustrate the conditions that some of these migrants experience.

CLINICAL CASES

Case 1: Clara

Clara is an 11-year-old American citizen of Salvadorian parents who had been raised in El Salvador since she was a toddler. She was referred to receive outpatient services by local Child Protective Services after her maternal aunt "dropped her off" in Imperial, California.

She spoke only Spanish, so she was scheduled with a bilingual therapist, who found out that she had witnessed the assassination of both her parents, who were shot in their car. It was suspected, although never confirmed, that her parents had been involved in criminal activities, as the only plausible explanation for being ambushed by "cocaleros," or cocaine traffickers. After this tragic event, she lived with her maternal grandmother, who died of natural causes a few months later. Her maternal aunt decided to bring her through Guatemala and Mexico, fleeing from the violence and poverty in their home country. Clara was separated from her aunt on entering the United States, because unlike Clara, the aunt was undocumented. Although they subsequently stayed in touch through sporadic phone calls, Clara had already experienced the loss of four of the most important people in her life; at the same time, she was trying to adapt to a "new" country, a new language, and a new culture.

On her first visit, Clara was properly groomed and dressed. She did not exhibit psychotic features. She was calm most of the time, but would break down crying intermittently because she was overwhelmed by the intrusive images that she would experience on a daily basis. She did not exhibit any suicidal or homicidal thoughts. She had no history of self-harm or risk-taking behaviors and no history of substance use.

During her therapy sessions, it became obvious that her mood was dysregulated as a result of the changing and chaotic attachment process experienced in the previous months. Fear of abandonment triggered her symptoms, making her fearful and scared. The event in which Clara witnessed her parents' assassination was imprinted into her psyche. The intensity of this event made it ever present and vivid, and with time, it started to become the only mental image left of her parents. Clara was diagnosed with PTSD. She was started on sertraline 25 mg/day to ameliorate the intensity of this traumatic memory.

As Clara sought comfort in her memories, she would only find the images of the tragedy, triggering once more the feelings of horror, fear, and loss that she experienced. She would cry, asking, "Why?," and would sob for long periods of time just repeating "mamita, mamita…" over and over again. With the image of her parents' gruesome deaths replacing almost all other images of her parents, Clara could not, or would not, let the image go.

The events required strong emotional containment, sometimes even surpassing the capacity of social services staff. This was one of the main reasons why Clara had experienced several changes in foster parents— once before starting treatment, and twice more while she was already in therapy: the foster parents would also be overwhelmed by her episodes and finally give up on her because they felt they could not help her. These changes in foster parents only added to the number of people who had "abandoned" her.

Therapy was prematurely stopped because Child Protective Services had located extended family out of state, where she was sent by the corresponding authorities.

Case 2: Virginia

Virginia is a 16-year-old Honduran citizen who entered Mexico illegally with the Via Crucis caravan while pregnant. Before making it into the United States, she was arrested for assaulting another female after an argument, while in the border city of Mexicali. Because of her age, she was placed at a shelter managed by local Child Protective Services, where she quickly exhibited defiant and verbally aggressive behavior, until she was transferred to a general hospital to give birth by cesarean section. On return to the shelter, her behavior worsened by becoming physically aggressive toward staff and peers, destroying objects, attempting to leave several times, and eventually threatening a staff member with a knife. The last action prompted an emergency evaluation and admission to a local acute psychiatric unit.

On admission, Virginia was irritable, verbally aggressive, defiant, and mostly uncooperative. There was no evidence of psychotic features or suicidal thoughts or plans. She reluctantly gave a history of symptoms compatible with depression. Virginia was diagnosed with major depressive disorder, recurrent, severe; and conduct disorder, childhood-onset type. She was started on a combination of fluoxetine and olanzapine, group therapy, and individual therapy.

During the ensuing days, she slowly opened up and was able to talk about her childhood. She recalled her mother dying when she was 5 and having no other relatives around. She was illiterate, having never went to school while growing up in the streets. She would work here and there cleaning houses, selling food, and even running errands for strangers. She started smoking tobacco at age 9 and through puberty used cannabis and methamphetamines, without an established pattern. She became sexually active at age 12 and, after several sexual partners, became pregnant by rape at age 13. The child who she gave birth to was taken away by local authorities. At age 15 she lived with an older man for a few months and became pregnant again, with the child she was carrying while in the caravan who was later born in Mexico. She described herself as prone to anger, and admitted getting into fights, stealing, and destroying property belonging to other people, either for pleasure or to "earn respect." She considered these behaviors not only normal but also fair and even necessary because of the environment where she grew up.

She further admitted to a history of depressed mood, crying spells, irritability, and a deep sense of guilt for several years. As the hospitalization progressed, her episodes of verbal and physical aggression decreased. She was described by nursing staff as manipulative and reluctantly cooperative with staff instructions. She became increasingly interested in reuniting with her baby, going back to school, and working at a decent job. Because of her migratory situation, and her being a minor and a mother, yet without family members, her future living conditions are up to Mexican authorities.

DISCUSSION

In this chapter we have attempted to give a brief description of the humanitarian crisis taking place at the UMBR, between the cities of Tijuana and San Diego, since the latter half of 2018. It has become evident that the Via Crucis caravan and its repercussions exceeded the capacity of the migration agencies in both countries, as they have been reacting with temporary, rather than long-term, solutions.

Selee et al. (2019), at the Migration Policy Institute (MPI), recognize as a positive step that the governments of the two countries have been in bilateral discussions to address the situation, while underscoring the urgent need to go beyond short-term migration control measures. They highlight the importance of implementing a different set of tools in order to outline the transition from irregular to legal migration. They especially emphasize the importance of preventing unintended consequences, such as strengthening the operations of migrant smugglers and reinforcing their ties to other organized crime networks (Selee et al. 2019).

Selee et al. (2019) also propose solutions in five areas that have been either unattended or poorly addressed:

1. *Improving the current asylum systems in both the United States and Mexico, which are insufficient and sluggish.* The most recent measures developed—the "remain in Mexico" policy and the newest one, a "safe third-country" agreement—are believed to endanger vulnerable migrants and to offer little in the way of timely protection. The proposal to remain in Mexico is of great concern because the current Mexican system faces enormous capacity issues, and the newest measure requires being denied asylum in the first country of transit before being able to request asylum in the United States. Selee et al. also recognize that there may be a mixture of motivations (e.g., economic, family reunification) and that not all cases are exclusively of people fleeing violent conditions, so they recommend ensuring fair but faster processing. They suggest this can be accomplished with better interviewing techniques, greater ability for officers to make final decisions, larger budgets, and the involvement of the United Nations. They further propose to process claims not only in the United States but also in Mexico and even in the countries of origin.

2. *Strengthening immigration institutions.* It is recommended that U.S. government officers more adequately handle families and minors, and that the Mexican government implement internal controls to prevent the alleged corruption and collusion between immigration officers and migrant smugglers.

3. *Targeting smuggling networks.* Preventing smuggling networks from operating will require sharing intelligence among the governments of key countries (i.e., Brazil, Ecuador, Panama, Costa Rica) in order to target the frontline smugglers, as well as their links to legal businesses (e.g., bus companies, hotels, restaurants) and other crime organizations, and incorporating strategies similar to those used to prevent narcotic smuggling.

4. *Creating a legal path to migration.* According to the MPI, research from previous migration movements has provided evidence that approaches such as work permits, deters illegal immigration and may persuade many would-be migrants to wait their turn.

5. *Investing in the countries of origin, for better and safer livelihoods.* Such efforts include addressing poverty as well as corruption, and, most importantly, having a clear idea of the needs and a clear plan of the desired structural changes, prior to making any investments (Clemens and Gough 2018; Selee et al. 2019).

The recommendations outlined above or similar recommendations may or may never be acted on. If they are, it may not be in the near future. Such decisions are clearly beyond the responsibility of mental health clinicians. Nonetheless, because of the nature of our work, we are likely to run into situations where we will have to address the needs of asylum seekers, along with potential language and cultural barriers, regardless of whether these recommendations ever get endorsed or not (Bustamante et al. 2017).

We have also presented two clinical vignettes of unfortunate victims of violent and underprivileged environments and described the repercussions of traumatic experiences to their mental health. Needless to say, these are individuals who one way or another were able to access psychiatric attention, one in the United States and the other one in Mexico. One can only wonder how many more asylum seekers in need are unable to access care, and how their symptoms, cognitive capacity, level of function, and ability to integrate to their new society might evolve.

Although the geopolitical, legal, financial, and trade issues surrounding these events remain in the field of anthropologists, economists, and other academicians, it is clear that mental health clinicians across the United States will sooner or later be exposed to patients affected by this phenomenon, because they were granted asylum and are getting established in this United States, they have a relative "stuck" in Mexico waiting for his or her application to be processed, or they lost someone to violence in their country of origin.

As to the migrants themselves, clinicians should keep in mind that there are at least three periods of potential exposure to trauma. Even though exposure does not always result in the development of PTSD, other disorders can be either exacerbated or triggered (i.e., conduct disorder, major depressive disorder). In the case of asylum seekers, who by definition are fleeing violent environments, exposure to trauma is present prior to beginning the migration process (premigration trauma); this is the first period in which trauma can occur and mental disorders triggered, and the main reason why asylum seekers decide to migrate. Once the migration process begins, asylum seekers remain at risk of trauma exposure as they transit to their desired destination (migration trauma). Once the migration process has been completed, regardless of whether asylum was granted or not, the process of adaptation and acculturation into the new environment represents a third period of potential trauma exposure (postmigration trauma) (Bustamante et al. 2017).

CONCLUSION

Seeking asylum into the United States and other economically developed countries is an ongoing phenomenon. It seems that various elements have come together since the dawn of the twenty-first century: an increased exodus from countries with civil and economic unrest, political overtones in the United States underscoring the inability and/or reluctance to continue granting asylum, and quick dispersal of the news across the globe via social media. This combination of elements is unique and has become a common topic of discussion and concern for the average citizen and resident in this country. Mental health professionals are not exempt from these concerns and are likely to elaborate their own set of beliefs and positions regarding the subject.

KEY CLINICAL POINTS

- Migrants seeking asylum, such as members of the Via Crucis caravan, are at risk of trauma-related disorders.
- Trauma exposure varies, as does its impact on the individual's health.
- Assessing for adverse childhood experiences is recommended in this vulnerable group.
- Usual treatments may have a reduced efficacy in trauma victims.
- Promotion of a safe environment is an essential part of the treatment plan.

REFERENCES

Altman CE, Gorman BK, Chávez S, et al: The mental well-being of Central American transmigrant men in Mexico. Glob Public Health 13(4):383–399, 2018 27185289

Associated Press: Trump's border wall prototypes demolished in San Diego. February 27, 2019. Available at: https://www.marketwatch.com/story/trumps-border-wall-prototypes-demolished-in-san-diego-2019-02-27. Accessed October 17, 2019.

Bustamante LHU, Cerqueira RO, Leclerc E, et al: Stress, trauma, and post-traumatic stress disorder in migrants: a comprehensive review. Br J Psychiatry 40(2):220–225, 2017 29069252

Carrillo G, Uribe F, Lucio R, et al: The United States-Mexico border environmental public health: the challenges of working with two systems. Rev Panam Salud Publica 41:e98, 2017 28902281

Castillo Udiarte R, Perez-Cruz E, Hidalgo-Vivas G, et al: Nadie me sabe dar razón. Tijuana: migración y memoria. Juarez, Mexico, Secretaría de Cultura, 2016

CBS News: US and Mexico reach last minute deal to avoid tariffs. June 8, 2019. Available at: https://www.cbsnews.com/news/trump-tariff-mexico-president-says-cancels-plan-after-deal-reached-on-immigration-today-2019-06-08/. Accessed October 17, 2019.

Clemens M, Gough K: Can regular migration channels reduce irregular migration? Lessons for Europe from the United States. February 2018. Available at: https://www.cgdev.org/sites/default/files/can-regular-migration-channels-reduce-irregular-migration.pdf. Accessed October 17, 2019.

CNN: State of the Union 2018. 2018. Available at: https://edition.cnn.com/2018/01/30/politics/2018-state-of-the-union-transcript/index.html. Accessed October 17, 2019.

Esténs MM: Life for migrants after the Via Crucis caravan to the US-Mexico border. May 22, 2018. Available at: https://indypendent.org/2018/05/life-for-migrants-after-the-via-crucis-caravan-to-the-u-s-mexico-border/. Accessed October 17, 2019.

Guild B: Government says Mexico border wall prototypes complete. CBS News, October 26, 2017. Available at: https://www.cbsnews.com/news/government-says-mexico-border-wall-prototypes-complete/. Accessed October 17, 2019.

Hernandez-Fuentes EJ, Ng B, Gonzalez-Hernandez IA: Methamphetamine and male suicide in the US-Mexico border region. OJIM 3:30–33, 2013

La Jeunesse W: Overwhelmed city asks Mexican government. Fox News, November 16, 2018. Available at: https://www.foxnews.com/world/as-migrant-caravan-reaches-tijuana-overwhelmed-city-asks-mexican-government-for-4-million. Accessed October 17, 2019.

Keller A, Joscelyne A, Granski M, et al: Pre-migration trauma exposure and mental health functioning among Central American migrants arriving at the US border. PLoS One 12(1):e0168692, 2017 28072836

Moore J, Almond K: This is what the US-Mexico border looks like. 2019. Available at: https://edition.cnn.com/interactive/2018/12/politics/border-wall-cnnphotos/. Accessed October 17, 2019.

Ng B, Ruiz P, Oquendo M, et al: Cultural issues on suicide, sociopathy, and opioids: an international Latino perspective. Council on International Psychiatry, Session 13412018. Presented at the annual meeting of the American Psychiatric Association, New York, NY, May 5–9, 2018

Partlow J, Miroff N: Deal with Mexico paves way for asylum overhaul at U.S. border. November 24, 2018. Available at: https://www.washingtonpost.com/world/national-security/deal-with-mexico-paves-way-for-asylum-overhaul-at-us-border/2018/11/24/87b9570a-ef74-11e8-9236-bb94154151d2_story.html?utm_term=.5b3fe3fc92f6. Accessed October 17, 2019.

Selee A, Giorguli-Saucedo SE, Masferrer C, et al: Strategic solutions for the United States and Mexico to manage the migration crisis. July 2019. Available at: https://www.migrationpolicy.org/news/strategic-solutions-united-states-and-mexico-manage-migration-crisis. Accessed October 17, 2019.

Specia M, Gladstone R: Border agents shot tear gas into Mexico. Was it legal? November 28, 2018. Available at: https://www.nytimes.com/2018/11/28/world/americas/tear-gas-border.html. Accessed October 17, 2019.

U.S. Customs and Border Protection: Southwest border migration FY 2019. September 9, 2019. Available at: https://www.cbp.gov/newsroom/stats/sw-border-migration. Accessed October 17, 2019.

U.S. Department of Health and Human Services: The US-Mexico border region. HHS.gov, December 13, 2017. Available at: https://www.hhs.gov/about/agencies/oga/about-oga/what-we-do/international-relations-division/americas/border-health-commission/us-mexico-border-region/index.html. Accessed October 17, 2019.

The White House: Executive order: border security and immigration enforcement improvements. January 25, 2017. Available at: https://www.whitehouse.gov/presidential-actions/executive-order-border-security-immigration-enforcement-improvements/. Accessed October 17, 2019.

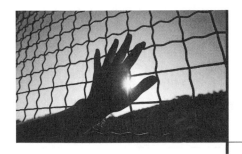

Chapter 11

TRAINING RESIDENTS TO TREAT REFUGEES

James Griffith, M.D.
Sara Teichholtz, M.D.

Providing care for a refugee can be the most complex but also among the most gratifying of clinical experiences. Care for a refugee requires cross-cultural skills for creating a therapeutic relationship across gaps of language and culture, often using an interpreter. It requires sufficient cultural humility so that one can be easily forgiven for mistakes and misunderstandings that inevitably occur. Grasping the emotional impact of displacement from one's home and categorical hatred based on ethnic identity requires a moral sensibility that extends beyond cultural competence. Psychiatric diagnosis and treatment of PTSD or major depressive disorder can be essential for relief of suffering due to traumatic stress. Yet most suffering that refugees experience is not due to mental illnesses, but rather to "normal suffering" from loss of a home, inadequate health care, lack of access to schooling for children, unsafe neighborhoods, or crowded living conditions. A psychiatrist has a dual mission

143

to provide care for both disorder and distress. All this is a demanding charge to give a psychiatry resident or other mental health trainee. Yet no other clinical encounter in all of psychiatry has so much to teach a psychiatrist about healing.

A Dual Mission: Strengthening Resilience While Treating Symptoms of Disorders

Treating a refugee should begin by responding to the refugee as a person, not as a patient. That is, one starts by meeting the refugee as a more-or-less normal human being affected by extreme and abnormal stressors, rather than as a patient with a mental illness. This normalizing attitude provides a frame of dignity within which a refugee can speak forthrightly about experiences of threat, violence, or humiliation that may feel difficult or shameful to put into words. A starting point is to learn first about the threatening circumstances that led to flight from the home country, including traumas and losses that occurred en route to sanctuary in the United States. This requires listening, understanding, and witnessing the person's accounts of loss, trauma, or dehumanization. After this personal story is understood and acknowledged, attention then can turn to diagnosis and treatment of psychiatric symptoms, such as depression or PTSD.

> Mr. B. was seeking political asylum in the United States after escaping imprisonment in Cameroon. The psychiatry resident asked Mr. B. what were his concerns that led to his visit to our clinic. Rather than answer this question, Mr. B. began telling his country's story of a long-standing dictatorship that student activists and opposition political parties sought to overcome through new multiparty elections in 1992. However, the authoritarian ruler suppressed his opposition in a flawed election, and Mr. B. and others were jailed and tortured. By the end of the first session, the psychiatry resident had only learned about the political history of Cameroon and was concerned that he perhaps should have pressed Mr. B. to stay on topic. His supervisor reassured the resident that Mr. B. wanted to know that his doctor understood the struggle that brought him to the United States before he would be comfortable entrusting the doctor with facts about his health. In subsequent sessions, Mr. B. did further describe his posttraumatic symptoms so that psychiatric treatment could be organized to treat them.

A simple maxim is to honor struggle. Ask first, "What happened to you?" before asking, "What is wrong with you?"

Focusing on a refugee's resilience is a reliable way to restore lost dignity. Questions should be asked about strengths, competencies, knowledge, or practical wisdom that helped that person prevail against harsh life conditions. Such questions include the following:

- What has kept you from giving up while facing so many hardships?
- What sustained hope during hard times?
- What are the strengths of your family that help you to stay strong?
- When going through hard times, to whom do you turn for help?
- Are there important religious beliefs or practices, or a religious community, that have helped you to endure?

Mr. M. was a refugee from a central African country who had escaped from prison when colleagues were able to bribe his jailors. He was seeking political asylum in the United States, but his wife and children remained in their home country.

"After all that you have endured, what has kept you from giving up?" the psychiatrist asked.

"My kids. I'm alive, and now I have to find work and help my kids. The school year is starting, and they will need money for school," he answered.

"Are there any people who help you?" the psychiatrist asked.

"Our pastor and the members of my church."

The psychiatry resident responded that finding work to enable him to help his children would be at the forefront of the refugee program's efforts. Mr. M. and the resident then planned a meeting with his church leaders to discuss how to solicit funds for his children's tuition. The resident also recommended an antidepressant for Mr. M.'s posttraumatic symptoms "to help you stay strong, and not to get worn down by poor sleep and intrusive memories, for the time when you will be reunited with your family."

Mr. M.'s response to a resilience question—What has kept you from giving up?—spoke to what mattered most for him (Griffith 2018). The different elements of subsequent treatment could then be organized around this central concern for his family. Eliciting strengths and mobilizing resources strengthened Mr. M.'s morale despite a lengthy list of adversities.

THE PSYCHIATRIC DIAGNOSTIC INTERVIEW

As discussed in earlier chapters, a psychiatric diagnostic interview with a refugee should assess in particular detail three domains of symptomatology associated with traumatic experiences, losses and grief, and acts of dehumanization, in addition to customary questions about social history, family history, medical history, and history of psychiatric illness or treatment.

TRAUMATIC EXPERIENCES

The key question is a version of "Did any events occur that should not ever happen to any person—such as assaults, abuse, or any other deliberately inflicted threats or pain?" Traumatic experiences occur when terror, horror, helplessness, or humiliation are present too intensely or for too long. The traumatic event persists as intrusive daytime memories or nighttime nightmares. Reminders of the event, such as sounds, smells, or images, may trigger physical sensations, shifts in mood, or intrusive images. Hearing loud or angry voices in the workplace, listening to news of war on television, or being exposed to an excess of lights and noise at a shopping mall all can become intolerable. Commonly, a traumatized person avoids such reminders, even to the extent of living a reclusive life.

Traumatic events typically have been the cause for a refugee's flight from a home country, but other traumatic events often have occurred during the journey to the United States or after arrival (Fernando et al. 2010; Miller et al. 2008; Rasmussen et al. 2010; Song et al. 2015). When traumatic events are acknowledged, an assessment instrument such as the Harvard Trauma Questionnaire may be useful for documenting the kinds and severity of traumatic events that occurred (Mollica et al. 1992). Beyond documenting occurrences of events, it is most important to learn how traumatic experiences continue to impact daily life functioning. Posttraumatic symptoms are often the cause of emotional pain, poor sleep, or difficulties in relationships or work. One can ask: "Are there ways in which the violent events that happened in the Sudan still affect your life now?" However, it can be of greater value to ask a refugee how he or she spends each hour of a typical day, from morning to night. This can help gauge the extent to which functioning in daily life is constricted by depressive or posttraumatic symptoms.

LOSSES AND GRIEF

Losses and consequent grief often constitute the greatest long-term impacts of violence that prompted the flight from a home country, even though posttraumatic symptoms may have predominated in the immediate aftermath (Keller et al. 2006; McKoll et al. 2008). Some refugees show depressive symptoms of such degree that a diagnosis of major depressive disorder (MDD) is warranted. MDD has characteristic symptoms, such as anhedonia, loss of self-regard, and suicidal ideation, that help distinguish it from demoralization and other normal syndromes of distress (Griffith and Norris 2012). High scores on validated quantitative mood assessment instruments, such as the Hamilton Depression Rating Scale (Hamilton 1960), can help distinguish MDD from other syndromes of distress.

ACTS OF DEHUMANIZATION

Refugees commonly have been treated inhumanely by discrimination, coercion, exploitation, violence, or torture based on their group of identity, whether it be religious, ethnic, racial, national, or political. These acts of social violence target group membership without regard to the suffering of victims as individual persons.

The emotional consequences of categorical hatred extend beyond symptoms of depression or PTSD. A broken sense of identity, loss of a capacity to trust others, self-loathing, and loss of empathy for one's own suffering can be other consequences. Individuals often suffer shame from internalized stigmatization (Agger 1994; Agger et al. 2012; Mollica 2006).

Psychotherapy for dehumanization requires a resilience orientation that focuses on what within the person is still intact and unsullied, beyond the reach of the abuser. A clinician can ask: "There is a place inside every person that evil cannot touch...Has there been a place like that within you? Can you tell me about it?" Bringing to the forefront those aspects of a person that defied the oppressor's assault provides a point of reference from which a stepwise program of recovery can begin.

An inventory should be taken of all that was taken away by the violence—whether home, family members, relationships, community, profession, or hopes for a good future—so that these losses can be fully acknowledged and respectfully mourned. The clinician should speak from the position of moral witness, stating explicitly that what happened was wrong, as in some version of "What happened to you was wrong, it was evil, and this should never happen to any person anywhere." Revenge against the abuser often can be framed as living well—that is, relearning to live well a life full of joy, meaningful relationships, and gratifying work (Mollica 2006; Weingarten 2000, 2010).

SKILL SETS OFTEN MISSING IN U.S. PSYCHIATRY RESIDENCIES

Treating refugees requires psychiatric skill sets that are not adequately taught in many U.S. psychiatry residencies. There are important differences between low- and middle-income countries and high-income countries in terms of ethnopsychologies, psychiatric diagnoses, morbidity of psychiatric illnesses, and social suffering. Standard curricula in U.S. psychiatry residencies may not provide certain skills needed for care of refugees who come to the United States from low- and middle-income countries (Griffith et al. 2016). Four skill sets that may require additional training through self-study and clinical workshops are discussed below.

DIAGNOSTIC AND TREATMENT METHODS FOR NORMAL SYNDROMES OF DISTRESS

Demoralization, grief, loss of identity, loss of dignity, and other forms of social suffering more often account for low mood states than does MDD as a psychiatric illness. Psychiatrists need skills for distinguishing this "normal suffering" from psychiatric illnesses. Demoralization, ambiguous loss, and loss of identity are three normal syndromes of distress that are particular sources of suffering for many refugees.

Demoralization

Demoralization refers to the helplessness, hopelessness, confusion, and subjective incompetence that people feel when sensing that they are failing their own or other's expectations for coping (Frank and Frank 2001). Demoralization is not a mental illness but rather a normal human response to circumstances perceived as overwhelming (Slavney 1999). An important distinction between demoralization and depression is that demoralized individuals display positive mood reactivity, in which their ability to experience hope and joy can be restored by good news, an unexpectedly positive turn of events, or a reduced burden of stressors. Demoralization, unlike depression, does not typically respond to antidepressant medication. Instead, it is important to acknowledge suffering, to honor struggle, to work with individuals to build on strengths and competencies, and to reduce the burden of stressors to the extent possible. Brief psychotherapeutic interventions have been designed for aiding persons coping with crises of demoralization (Catapano and Griffith 2019; Griffith 2018; Griffith and Gaby 2005).

> Mr. A. was a teacher in a university in a West African country when he was arrested for participating in a demonstration protesting corrupt university officials who were financially exploiting students. Mr. A. was beaten by police, deprived of sleep, and subjected to lengthy interrogations. After release from prison, threats and police surveillance continued until family advised him to leave the country to seek asylum in the United States Although he was granted asylum in the United States, he felt

isolated and unable to find employment except in a retail store. He lost hope that he would ever regain an academic career. At his primary care clinic, his physician requested psychiatric consultation to treat Mr. A.'s depression. The psychiatry resident noted that Mr. A. was able to enjoy pleasurable activities. His Hamilton Depression Rating Scale score was only mildly elevated, despite his distress. The psychiatry resident explained to Mr. A. that he appeared demoralized, not depressed, and that the distress he was experiencing was "what most anyone would feel given what you are going through." The resident then focused his interview on two themes: first, identifying strengths and skills that Mr. A. had relied on when coping with past adversities so these could be applied to his current challenges, and, second, clarifying the values that Mr. A. had expressed by confronting corruption on behalf of his students in order to honor his courage. The psychiatrist discussed with Mr. A. how he could best mobilize his signature strengths in his current life situation, how he could continue to express his deepest values in his new life setting, and how he could begin organizing a social network he could rely upon. No medication was prescribed.

Ambiguous Loss

Ambiguous loss is a kind of loss that is keenly felt but is unwitnessed by other people not sharing the experience (Boss 1999). Ambiguous loss is a common feature of a refugee's experience in a new country, when absence of the old country may be what is most present in a refugee's awareness but not visible to others. A normal loss, such as bereavement after a death, follows a normal course of expectable grief and in time finds closure. Ambiguous loss, however, has no clear boundaries and can be difficult to resolve. Because it receives no validation from others, an individual with ambiguous loss may have difficulty managing the distress while receiving no social support.

Ambiguous loss includes the loss of meaning that many political activists experience after gaining asylum in the United States. They are now physically safe but in a kind of meaningless purgatory within a new country that has no awareness of the human rights struggles they fought or the losses they endured in their home country. As a Latin American refugee in Denmark commented:

> In my homeland, I was very involved. I had a dream. It was as if my life had meaning, and it wasn't something individual. But here in Denmark, I only decide for myself. If you don't have any cause, any individual dream— it is no longer collective. And of course, I also have children, and I think about their future. But we human beings need a dream, a goal for our lives, for otherwise life has no meaning. (Agger 1994, p. 125)

Ambiguous loss can be addressed by naming ambiguity, not the ambiguous situation, as the primary problem (Griffith and Griffith 2002, pp. 292–297). In dialogues with the clinician, losses can be acknowledged fully and spoken about. How to deal with the ambiguity can itself be the focus of a treatment session. It often is useful to engage the family as a whole in acknowledging and discussing ambiguous losses.

> Mr. H. was a young man when the Taliban seized Mazar-e Sharif, the region of Afghanistan where he was living with his family. In less than a week, the Taliban killed thousands of individuals, including many members of Mr. H.'s extended family. He fled Afghanistan with his wife and children and gained political asylum in the United States but leaving behind the rest of his extended family. Memories of the difficulties moving to the United States with its different culture and language have faded over the years. However, the memories of his traumatic experiences in Afghanistan remain with him. An antidepressant and prazosin for nightmares reduced the severity of his PTSD symptoms. He now lives within an Afghan refugee community of 45,000, and his children have successfully navigated the U.S. educational system and live productive adult lives. Yet Mr. H. feels a sadness that is unending. He continuously misses the conversations of old friends and the countryside of Afghanistan from which he is absent. Each year he suffers a recurrence of profound grief upon the anniversary of the fall of Mazar-e Sharif. His clinicians and case manager each year acknowledge his grief and listen to his recollections of family life in the Mazar-e Sharif countryside before the Taliban came.

Loss of Identity

Migration to a new country commonly is accompanied by a drop in socioeconomic status, loss of profession, and losses of other community or societal roles. Such losses of identity can be a part of ambiguous loss and a cause of demoralization. Salman Akhtar (2011) has described four factors—separation from familiar topography, loss of personal possessions, alteration of man-animal relationships, and encounters with the new physical objects—that generate anxiety and mourning because of their impacts on identity. Maladaptive responses include a repudiation that denies the changes, as in a fantasy of return to their home even if unsafe or unrealistic, or re-creating a semblance of their old home in their new location.

Even though the interdisciplinary role of a psychiatry resident is often psychopharmacological management of posttraumatic and mood symptoms, time remaining in a treatment session after checking symptoms and side effects can be used to listen, acknowledge, and witness a refugee's struggle to grieve losses. These conversations can help a refugee to discern what to hold onto from old identities and what new changes to embrace.

> Dr. D. had been a surgeon in his former Middle Eastern country. Although political asylum in the United States provided safety, he was aware he would never practice medicine again because of the practical impossibility of gaining medical licensure. Further, the human rights advocacy for which he had put his life at risk in his former society had no context in the United States that would continue to give it meaning. Treatment sessions with his psychiatry resident focused on not only his PTSD symptoms but also dialogues about daily life and possible new directions to consider. After a long period of sorrow and discouragement, Dr. D. completed a master's degree program to become a licensed professional counselor in an addiction treatment center. Although his path as a physician was blocked, he nevertheless found a meaningful role as a healer.

FAMILY-CENTERED PSYCHIATRIC CARE

In many cultures, a person's primary identity is that of a family member, not that of an individual. This social unit extends beyond the nuclear family to include the extended family with grandparents, aunts, uncles, and cousins. Effective treatment often must engage the family unit, not only the individual patient. Family therapy skills are needed for working with refugees' families as the primary unit of care (Griffith and Keane 2018; Griffith et al. 2016). These skills include establishing a therapeutic alliance with the family as a whole, providing family psychoeducation, arriving at a systemic formulation of clinical problems, and developing action plans that involve multiple family members.

> Ms. Q. was an elderly matriarch in an Arabic family from the Middle East. Psychiatric consultation was sought by her primary care physician because of her depressed mood. She was spending her day sitting alone silently. An inquiry into her family life revealed how she had devoted her life to parenting her three sons, making extensive personal sacrifices that had included work outside the home for extra income. Now adults, her sons had successfully completed their educations and found employment in another city. Ms. Q.'s husband mostly stayed in his room. The psychiatry resident convened a meeting of all family members to discuss how the family could be helpful in Ms. Q.'s care. A family intervention was designed that included scheduled visits by the sons, Ms. Q.'s husband accompanying her to medical visits for her diabetes, and pro scription of an antidepressant medication.

ETHNOPHARMACOLOGY

Ethnic differences are associated with differences in the effects of medications, largely due to dietary/genetic influences on drugs (Lin et al. 1993; Ruiz 2000). Most psychiatric drugs undergo metabolism in the liver by enzymes of the cytochrome P450 system, particularly the 1A2, C19, 2D6, and 34A enzymes. The efficiency of 2D6 drug metabolism varies according to the genetic ancestry of different ethnic groups. The 2D6 enzyme system has a major role in determining how rapidly many antidepressant and typical antipsychotic medications are metabolized. "Super metabolizers" have multiple copies of the enzyme and can metabolize medications much more quickly than others, so that drug levels remain quite low and medications are less effective. This can lead a clinician to an incorrect judgment that the patient is not taking the medication. Up to 30% of Ethiopians, 19% of Saudi Arabians, and 10% of Spanish individuals are super metabolizers. "Slow metabolizers," in contrast, have enzyme systems that are less efficient at metabolizing medications, causing increased levels of medications at normal doses. Up to 35% of Nicaraguans, 35%–50% of African Americans, 35% of Asians, and 3% of Mexican Americans are slow metabolizers. 2D6 enzymes are also influenced by diet, with high corn diets slowing metabolism. Other enzyme systems can be induced or inhibited by dietary factors such as grapefruit juice, coffee, watercress, alcohol, cabbage, carrots, and high protein diets (Chen et al. 2008; Wong and Pi 2012).

> Ms. T. was a 40-year old refugee from Ethiopia. Psychiatric consultation was requested by her psychotherapist because of worsening depression despite treatment with fluoxetine 40 mg daily. Ms. T. previously had been treated with sertraline, but with little improvement. The psychiatry resident was aware that a third of Ethiopians are cytochrome 2D6 "super metabolizers" and that this could possibly affect metabolism of both sertraline and fluoxetine. The resident changed Ms. T.'s antidepressant medication to citalopram 20 mg daily, because citalopram is metabolized by the 2C19 enzyme system and not the 2D6. Her depression symptoms began improving during the second week of citalopram treatment.

HUMAN RIGHTS ADVOCACY AS A ROUTINE ELEMENT OF PSYCHIATRIC CARE

Promoting mental health for refugees often entails political activism to address inequities in mental health policies and access to services. Whereas attention is usually paid to premigration stressors, the new country experience is often implicated in harm to a refugee's mental health. Stigma, discrimination, hostility, and physical violence in the new country are all factors that have an impact on the experience of postresettlement. In Scotland, the Sanctuary program has sought to understand the mental health experiences of asylum seekers and refugees. It found that many refugees felt they had swapped the stress of living in a war-torn or impoverished country with new stresses of uncertainty and isolation that were equivalent in magnitude, particularly fears of detention and deportation (Quinn et al. 2011). This study emphasized the need to confront institutional discrimination experienced by the asylum seeker and refugee communities.

> Ms. N. was a young woman from Uganda who had fled her home country after severe sexual abuse by a relative that had gone unrecognized by her family. She sought treatment for symptoms of PTSD and depression, for which medication was prescribed by her psychiatry resident. However, her greatest concern was the stress of uncertainty about her asylum application. Her mood and PTSD symptoms fluctuated with her level of fear that she might be forced to return home. As the political rhetoric about immigration policies grew heated, her fears of deportation intensified to the point that she would hide in her home should anyone knock on her door unexpectedly, fearing that it would be the police. The resident worked with her to distinguish anxiety from realistic fears, adopting different strategies for each.

The "seven D's"—discrimination, detention, dispersal, destitution, denial of health care, delayed decisions, and denial of the right to work—indicate specific points where advocacy and political activism can be addressed in the host country to reduce adverse impacts of postmigration stressors (McKoll et al. 2008). By targeting these points alongside clinical care, psychiatrists can play critical roles in advocacy for refugees.

> Ms. C. was a 44-year-old refugee from a West African country whose asylum petition was denied. She was ordered deported by an Immigration and Naturalization Service (INS) judge. Rather than report for deportation, she instead found employment as a nurse's aide and eventually completed her nursing education for a certificate degree. She was provided care in a community-based torture treatment program for chronic PTSD caused by detainment, beatings, and sexual assault by police in her home country due to her political activities. As her new life stabilized, she was unexpectedly arrested and detained for 2 years in an INS facility. When the torture treatment program learned about her detention, a psychiatric consultant, supported by a pro bono law firm, successfully

argued that her new onset of hallucinations, delusions, and suicidal impulses was due to the adverse conditions of the detainment center. She was released to live in her community with monthly reporting to an INS center. When her new attorneys reviewed her case, they discovered that the original INS judge had refused the report of an expert psychiatrist witness to be admitted as evidence. They appealed her case to an appellate court, which found the initial judge to have been in error. The appellate court ordered that her appeal for asylum be conducted again and with acceptance of expert testimony. Using a verbatim transcript of the initial trial, the psychiatric consultant, as expert witness, illustrated how Ms. C.'s errors in memory of events were most plausibly explained by the patient's severity of PTSD symptoms. On the basis of this testimony, the judge granted her asylum. The duration in time from initial court hearing to the awarding of asylum was 10 years.

CONCLUSION

Providing care for a refugee is a complex but gratifying experience for a psychiatrist. It often expands a psychiatrist's repertoire of clinical skills through its focus on assessment and care for normal syndromes of distress, ethnopharmacology, family-centered care, and human rights advocacy. It teaches how to conduct a resilience-building approach to treatment.

Providing care for a refugee teaches about both the harm done and the recovery possible when a psychiatrically healthy person is subjected to intentional violence. Unlike most psychiatric patients, a refugee typically is without genetic risks or early-life emotional injuries that otherwise would have set the course for psychiatric illness. A refugee typically would never be in the mental health system except that egregious threats or violence were visited on an otherwise normal human being. As such, it compels a treating psychiatrist to come to grips with moral issues in psychiatric treatment—a discourse about good and evil, justice and injustice, guilt and atonement. Providing care for a refugee becomes an opportunity not only to treat symptoms of illness but to restore humanity to a person who has been disinherited.

KEY CLINICAL POINTS

- Treating refugees is a complicated task for which residents in most training programs have little experience.
- The treatment needs to focus on resilience to restore lost dignity.

- Residents need to learn about the common syndromes of PTSD and depression but also of refugee demoralization, with its confusion and its subjective feelings of incompetence.

- Understanding ambiguous loss—loss that is felt but unwitnessed by others—is a theme to be addressed.

- Loss of identity occurs as refugees enter a new country with changes in economic status, friendships, and even language.

- Although medicine has a significant role to play in treatment of refugees, the unique factors of demoralization, ambiguous loss, and loss of identity need to be learned by residents in training. Clearly, supervisors need to have experience and skills to train residents in these activities.

REFERENCES

Agger I: The Blue Room: Trauma and Testimony Among Refugee Women— A Psycho-Social Exploration. Translated by Bille M. London, Zed Books, 1994

Agger I, Igreja V, Kiehle R, et al: Testimony ceremonies in Asia: integrating spirituality in testimonial therapy for torture survivors in India, Sri Lanka, Cambodia, and the Philippines. Transcult Psychiatry 49(3–4):568–589, 2012 22637721

Akhtar S: The trauma of geographic dislocation, Immigration and Acculturation: Mourning, Adaptation, and the Next Generation. New York, Jason Aronson, 2011, pp 3–30

Boss P: Ambiguous Loss: Learning to Live With Unresolved Grief. Cambridge, MA, Harvard University Press, 1999

Catapano L, Griffith JL: Building resilience and mobilizing hope in brief psychotherapy, in Mental Health and Illness Worldwide: Education About Mental Health and Illness. Edited by Pi EH, Hoon TC, Hermans MHM. New York, Springer, 2018, pp 345–372

Chen CH, Chen CY, Lin KM: Ethnopsychopharmacology. Int Rev Psychiatry 20(5):452–459, 2008 19012131

Fernando GA, Miller KE, Berger DE: Growing pains: the impact of disaster-related and daily stressors on the psychological and psychosocial functioning of youth in Sri Lanka. Child Dev 81(4):1192–1210, 2010 20636690

Frank JD, Frank JB: Persuasion and Healing: A Comparative Study of Psychotherapy, 3rd Edition. Baltimore, MD, Johns Hopkins University Press, 2001, p. 14

Griffith JL: Hope modules: brief psychotherapeutic interventions to counter demoralization from daily stressors of chronic illness. Acad Psychiatry 42(1):135–145, 2018 28752229

Griffith JL, Gaby L: Brief psychotherapy at the bedside: countering demoralization from medical illness. Psychosomatics 46(2):109–116, 2005 15774948

Griffith JL, Griffith ME: Engaging the Sacred in Psychotherapy: How to Talk With People About Their Spiritual Lives. New York, Guilford Press, 2002, pp. 292–297.

Griffith JL, Keane J: Where is the family in global mental health? Fam Syst Health 36(2):144–147, 2018 29902031

Griffith JL, Norris L: Distinguishing spiritual, psychological, and psychiatric issues in palliative care: Their overlap and differences. Prog Palliat Care 20:79–85, 2012

Griffith JL, Kohrt B, Dyer A, et al: Training psychiatrists for global mental health: cultural psychiatry, collaborative inquiry, and ethics of alterity. Acad Psychiatry 40(4):701–706, 2016 27060095

Hamilton M: A rating scale for depression. J Neurol Neurosurg Psychiatry 23:56–62, 1960 14399272

Keller A, Lhewa D, Rosenfeld B, et al: Traumatic experiences and psychological distress in an urban refugee population seeking treatment services. J Nerv Ment Dis 194(3):188–194, 2006 16534436

Lin K-M, Poland RE, Nakasaki G: Psychopharmacology and Psychobiology of Ethnicity. Progress in Psychiatry Series #39. Washington, DC, American Psychiatric Press, 1993, pp 61–186

McKoll H, McKenzie K, Bhui K: Mental healthcare of asylum-seekers and refugees. Adv Psychiatr Treat 14:452–459, 2008

Miller KE, Omidian P, Rasmussen A, et al: Daily stressors, war experiences, and mental health in Afghanistan. Transcult Psychiatry 45(4):611–638, 2008 19091728

Mollica RF: Healing Invisible Wounds: Paths to Hope and Recovery in a Violent World. New York, Harcourt, 2006

Mollica RF, Caspi-Yavin Y, Bollini P, et al: The Harvard Trauma Questionnaire. Validating a cross-cultural instrument for measuring torture, trauma, and posttraumatic stress disorder in Indochinese refugees. J Nerv Ment Dis 180(2):111–116, 1992 1737972

Quinn N, Shirjeel S, Siebelt L, et al: An Evaluation of the Sanctuary Community Conversation Programme to Address Mental Health Stigma With Asylum Seekers and Refugees in Glasgow. Glasgow, Scotland, NHS Health Scotland, 2011

Rasmussen A, Nguyen L, Wilkinson J, et al: Rates and impact of trauma and current stressors among Darfuri refugees in Eastern Chad. Am J Orthopsychiatry 80(2):227–236, 2010 20553516

Ruiz P (ed): Psychopharmacology in the Context of Culture and Ethnicity (Review of Psychiatry Series, Vol 19; Oldham JM and Riba MB, series eds.). Washington, DC, American Psychiatric Press, 2000, pp 1–36

Slavney PR: Diagnosing demoralization in consultation psychiatry. Psychosomatics 40(4):325–329, 1999 10402879

Song SJ, Kaplan C, Tol WA, et al: Psychological distress in torture survivors: pre- and post-migration risk factors in a US sample. Soc Psychiatry Psychiatr Epidemiol 50(4):549–560, 2015 25403567

Weingarten K: Witnessing, wonder, and hope. Fam Process 39(4):389–402, 2000 11143594

Weingarten K: Reasonable hope: construct, clinical applications, and supports. Fam Process 49(1):5–25, 2010 20377632

Wong FK, Pi EH: Ethnopsychopharmacology considerations for Asians and Asian Americans. Asian J Psychiatr 5(1):18–23, 2012 26878942

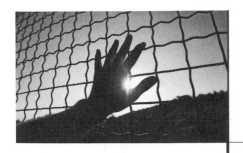

Chapter 12

ETHICAL CHALLENGES CONFRONTING PSYCHIATRISTS IN THE FIELD OF REFUGEE MENTAL HEALTH

Derrick Silove, A.M., M.B. Ch.B. (Hons I), M.D., FRANZCP, FASSA

Psychiatrists in the refugee mental health field encounter a range of ethical issues, as may be expected when working with a population that has been exposed to the most extreme forms of injustice and that in many circumstances continue to experience ongoing discrimination and exclusion. The nature of the refugee experience invariably results in a

The author wishes to thank Mr. Louis Klein, Senior Research Officer in the Psychiatry Research and Teaching Unit, for his invaluable assistance in preparing the manuscript.

blurring between the considerations of clinical ethics, which focuses primarily on the doctor-patient relationship, and the broader human rights domain that extends to the relationship of the individual and group to the state. In making a comprehensive assessment of the ethical issues involved, therefore, it is useful to adopt a multisystem framework that takes into account influences at the individual, family, group, and, at times, state and international levels.

This chapter provides examples of ethical dilemmas confronted at overlapping levels in the multisystem framework. Primary attention will be given to the clinical setting in which most psychiatrists spend the majority of their time. At a statewide level, the practice of prolonged detention of asylum seekers will be used to illustrate the ethical dilemmas encountered in settings where national policies have a direct impact on the human rights and mental health of displaced persons. Finally, reference will be made to the ethical responsibilities of psychiatrists when engaging in public debate concerning global issues that are critical to the rights and well-being of refugees, in this instance, arising from the tension between defending cultural rights as opposed to the right to accessing mental health services. The overarching objective throughout the chapter is to provoke thought and reflection rather than to offer definitive answers to complex questions. Although universal principles of ethics provide a guide, each challenge has unique aspects requiring a fresh analysis, and often serial reanalysis, in which the practitioner draws on multiple sources of knowledge and assistance. These include the established principles and guidelines established by precedent and adopted by professional bodies; the available literature on the relevant topic; the psychiatrist's personal moral values and belief systems; and, most importantly, access to the advice of trusted peers and mentors.

THE PSYCHIATRIST-PATIENT RELATIONSHIP WITHIN A CLINICAL SERVICE SETTING

Entry into the field of refugee mental health poses immediate challenges to the novice psychiatrist. As a member of society, the psychiatrist is exposed to highly charged representations and images of refugees that can oscillate between two extremes: at times refugees are welcomed as heroes who deserve society's compassion and generosity, whereas at other times this minority can be portrayed as intruders who present a threat to the integrity and stability of the host society. In contemporary times many societies appear to be polarized on this issue. In politically charged environments, the term *refugee* itself can be used in a pejorative and discriminatory manner, especially if it is affixed to the person as a permanent label—a process of reification that psychiatrists and other mental health professionals should be active in discouraging. In general, therefore, psychiatrists need to be vigilant to even subtle influences that public representations of refugees can exert on their responses and practices.

At the other extreme is the risk that newcomers to the field of practice will idealize their refugee patients, especially those who have been political activists striving for the defense of just causes in their home countries. Inexperienced therapists therefore may be overzealous in their efforts to assist patients, often by trying to do too much in too short a time. Overinvolvement can encourage dependency in the patient that undermines a primary goal of therapy, which is to promote autonomy and empowerment, which for refugees is fundamental to both the recovery process and successful acculturation to the new society. Skilled supervision for newcomers to the field can assist the novice to establish a balance between compassion and dispassion, providing active practical assistance and promoting independence in their patients.

The emergence of a specialist field of refugee mental health runs the risk of inadvertently discouraging general psychiatrists from engaging with refugees on the basis of the false premise that they lack the skills to do so. It is important to reverse that perception, given the large number of refugees in need of treatment worldwide. Generalists should be assured that applying first principles of practice goes a long way in treating refugees with common mental disorders. Psychiatrists can gain the additional knowledge they need by consultation with specialists and by undertaking their own research to familiarize themselves with the culture, customs, and history of individual refugee groups. By showing a willingness to learn from patients about their culture and history, psychiatrists demonstrate their respect and regard for the person as a source of knowledge and experience, which in turn serves to deepen and strengthen the therapeutic alliance.

Maintaining confidentiality and privacy can present special challenges in the refugee field. This is particularly true when interpreters are used, given that they often originate from the same background as the refugee, or in some instances in the same community, when the community is small or geographically concentrated, as is often the case in resettlement countries (i.e., interpreters may be known to the patient or to the family). At the extreme, it is possible that the interpreter is associated with an opposing faction in a past internecine conflict. If a problem is suspected, separate discussions with the interpreter and the patient may resolve the issue, especially if the patient does not object to working with the interpreter. In the discussion, however, the psychiatrist needs to be alert to the possibility that patients from traditional cultures may be compliant because of the customary respect shown to doctors or may be reluctant to raise concerns because of adverse past experiences in relating to government institutions including health services.

Most modern services in refugee mental health adopt a multidisciplinary model in which patients engage with a range of practitioners and personnel—for example, for general health needs, physiotherapy, work preparation, language classes, and family interventions. In these settings, there can be inadvertent breaches of confidentiality in relation to sensitive personal details during the process of communication between practitioners and agencies. Establishing clear service policies and ensuring their implementation through training and supervision are important provisions to avert transgressions of this type. Preserving confidentiality can also be made more difficult when, as is often the case, multiple members of the family attend the same mental health service. Customs relating to confidentiality and privacy at the family level differ across cultures and religious groups. For example, in patriarchal societies, husbands may expect to be apprised of any disclosures made by the wife to the doctor, and in some instances may insist on being present at all consultations with the partner. While sensitive to these cultural expectations, psychiatrists need to remain steadfast in adhering to contemporary professional codes governing confidentiality and privacy, and patients and their families need to be informed of these provisions.

A confronting issue for the psychiatrist that has received little attention in the refugee literature arises when a patient is found to be a perpetrator of human rights abuses. This possibility is particularly high when working among refugees who were combatants in regions of irregular warfare in which civilians were a major target. Male ex-combatants may have been implicated in the mass rape of women, and refugees who were young at the time may have been child soldiers forced to enact gross human rights violations, often against their own kin and families. Torturers may use the guise of being refugees to escape capture and indictment, and in some instances these persons present to mental health services in host countries.

Psychiatrists are likely to experience a mixture of personal and professional responses to uncovering perpetrators in their ongoing practice. In most situations, with the help of supervisors or mentors, the psychiatrist is able to continue with the therapy. Nevertheless, in some cases, the actions of the patient may be so abhorrent to the therapist that after careful deliberation and consultation with colleagues and supervisors, it is deemed appropriate to refer him or her elsewhere. An added complexity is that there may be grounds for indictment of patients according to human rights law, a situation in which confidentiality cannot be preserved and the patient needs to be informed that the practitioner is required to seek appropriate legal advice.

The psychiatrist also faces specific ethical issues when intimate partner violence is identified or suspected. Detection of the problem, which commonly is hidden, is an important responsibility requiring a high level of vigilance on the part of the treating psychiatrist. For example, intimate partner violence may be the hidden source of chronic depression among women refugees who are not responding to conventional treatments (Rees et al. 2016). It is not uncommon for the perpetrator to be a past advocate of human rights who was tortured for his opposition to an oppressive regime. Aggression at home in these cases often is a direct outcome of a posttraumatic stress reaction in which impulsive anger is a major feature. In these circumstances, perpetrators often experience intense feelings of guilt and shame, given their strong background values regarding the defense of human rights. In other situations, the pathways to intimate partner violence are not as clear-cut—for example, when patriarchal values, a sense of male entitlement, or tensions in the family relating to gender role changes in the new society are contributors to domestic conflict (Rees et al. 2018).

In all cases in which intimate partner violence is detected, the first responsibility of the psychiatrist is to ensure effective protection for the woman (and when necessary, her children)—a mandatory requirement in many host societies. The imperative to take action needs to be explained to both members of the couple. For some male perpetrators, revealing the problem can be a source of relief, especially when their violent behavior is felt to be ego-dystonic. In that sense, the identification of intimate partner violence may be a turning point in therapy for both the patient and the family. However, other situations may be much more complex and require involvement of a range of agencies with specialist roles in dealing with violence in the home.

Flexibility in the approach taken in psychotherapy with refugees experiencing traumatic stress reactions is not simply a technical but also an ethical issue. In that regard, the contemporary literature on psychotherapy in the refugee field can be misleading—particularly to the extent that it promotes the notion that a brief cognitive-behavioral therapy in which systematic exposure to trauma memories represents a central and essential component is the treatment of choice (Neuner et al. 2004). The reality is that some survivors of extreme trauma, particularly torture, can be overwhelmed if they are induced to confront memories of their trauma directly, at least early in therapy. Putting pressure on survivors to engage in exposure therapy can worsen symptoms and lead to adverse consequences including loss of control over aggressive impulses and alcohol abuse. In that regard, adherence by the psychiatrist to the first principle of ethics, which is to do no harm (*primum non nocere*), is of paramount importance. When the therapist is judging which therapy is most appropriate and safe, each refugee patient needs to be assessed carefully in relation to his or her strengths, vulnerabilities, capabilities, and preferences. Technical preferences by the therapist for a particular modality of therapy should never take precedence over an assessment of the risks involved in pursuing a particular approach.

Finally, psychiatrists in the refugee field have a special responsibility to maintain their own mental health. No practitioner is immune to the emotional and moral challenges encountered in everyday practice with refugee populations exposed to extreme human rights violations. Paradoxically, the sense of commitment and responsibility felt by psychiatrists to their patients can discourage them from recognizing the need for personal respite from the cumulative stress of working in the field. As a consequence, psychiatrists may ignore signs of early burn-out in themselves, even when changes in their behavior are obvious to colleagues, family, and, at times, patients. Psychiatrists have a duty to communicate their concerns to a colleague should they suspect that he or she is experiencing early features of burn-out. For all personnel working in the field, active strategies of self-care are imperative and should be encouraged by the service in which they work.

ETHICS AT THE INSTITUTIONAL LEVEL: ETHICAL RESPONSIBILITIES OF PSYCHIATRISTS IN RESPONDING TO POLICIES OF DETERRENCE APPLIED TO ASYLUM SEEKERS

As indicated, clinical practice in the refugee field cannot be separated from society-wide influences, including national immigration policies. Over recent decades, refugee recipient nations of the West have drawn a sharp distinction between refugees granted permanent residency prior to arrival in the country and asylum seekers who enter the host country without authorized resettlement visas. Increasingly, asylum seekers are being confined for indefinite periods in detention centers in prisonlike conditions even though they have not committed any crime. In that regard, the tendency to label asylum seekers as illegal immigrants to justify harsh policies aimed at deterring their arrival runs counter to the principles of international covenants such as the Universal Declaration of Human Rights and the United Nations Convention Related to the Status of Refugees. These instruments make it clear that seeking asylum as a refuge from persecution is a right not a crime.

Australia has taken a lead role in detaining asylum seekers, a polic‑ that was commenced in the late 1980s. At first, detention centers were built around the country, including in remote regions, but more recently, asylum seekers have been transferred to facilities on the neighboring Pacific Island countries of Nauru and Papua New Guinea. Several concerns have been raised repeatedly about conditions in detention, including the monotonous, regimented, prisonlike environments; the lack of schooling and play facilities for children; the inadequacy of medical and psychiatric services; and the periodic exposure of inmates to episodes of violence, including riots, burning of facilities, protests, and confrontations with guards.

From the outset, a small group of Australian psychiatrists played an active role in supporting asylum seekers by providing direct clinical services to detainees, writing legal reports in support of refugee claims, undertaking research, and offering expert testimony at a series of national and international inquiries into the human rights issues involved. The message has remained consistent: prolonged detention—a substantial number of refugees have been held for over 5 years—can retraumatize asylum seekers and exacerbate preestablished traumatic stress disorders. Early observations of this retraumatizing effect were evident to psychiatrists treating detainees, and these impressions were reinforced by an insider account by a detained Iraqi doctor, in an article published in the leading medical journal in Australia, in which the stages of despair and depression manifested by long-term inmates were vividly described (Sultan and O'Sullivan 2001). At the time, the government rejected claims that prolonged detention could cause psychological harm, partly on the basis that there was no systematic evidence to support these assertions. Yet, approaches by psychiatrists to undertake research in immigration detention centers were either ignored or declined.

After overcoming significant institutional and political barriers, a team at the University of New South Wales (UNSW) School of Psychiatry and collaborators completed a number of studies among asylum seekers both in the community and in detention. In one study, phone interviews were conducted by same-language psychologists with a group of detained families held in a remote detention center, a process facilitated by lawyers and volunteer visitors (Steel et al. 2004). A further study examined the longer-term effects of prolonged confinement on detainees released on temporary protection visas (Steel et al. 2006). On the basis of these and subsequent studies in other countries, key inferences could be drawn: that detained asylum seekers, including children, exhibited unusually high rates of PTSD, depression, and anxiety; that the traumas and stressors experienced in detention played a major role in perpetuating these symptoms; and that psychiatric disturbances tended to persist in ex-detainees for years after release into the community (noting that by far the majority of detainees in Australia are ultimately found to be genuine refugees). These findings formed the basis of psychiatric testimony presented to a succession of inquiries, including an inquiry by the Australian Human Rights Commission—hearings that repeatedly concluded that prolonged detention was detrimental to the mental health and well-being of asylum seekers, especially children (Australian Human Rights Commission 2014).

Nevertheless, individual psychiatrists in Australia challenged both the validity of the findings and the ethics of undertaking research among detainees. In one instance, the government engaged a psychiatrist to examine the scientific validity of the studies undertaken by the UNSW team. Ultimately, the rigor and legitimacy of the research were fully vindicated, but only after a painstaking inquiry that incurred great cost in time and effort for the research team. Thereafter, in a special series on the topic, an article was published in an Australian bioethical journal in which the author, a psychiatrist who had worked with government in relation to transcultural mental health policy and practice, claimed that the research undertaken by colleagues in detention centers was unethical because it put inmates at risk (Minas 2004; see also Steel and Silove 2004). A rejoinder by an independent group of psychiatrists and ethicists from a leading center in transcultural psychiatry in Canada took a contrary view, arguing that psychiatrists have an overriding responsibility to reveal human rights transgressions and their impact on the mental health of vulnerable populations, especially in institutions that are closed to public scrutiny and as long as participants are aware of the risks involved and give informed consent (Kirmayer et al. 2004). As it turned out, asylum seeker families participating in the study in question were released soon after the data were made public, most likely because of the compelling nature of the findings (Steel et al. 2006).

These events indicate the risks involved when psychiatrists are pitted against one another in politically and ethically charged situations such as in the midst of the public debate concerning asylum detention in Australia. What is perhaps unique about the history of this issue in Australia is that in spite of the constraints encountered, psychiatrists and other mental health professionals pursued the task of gathering evidence to support claims of harm being caused to asylum seekers held in prolonged detention. As such, the inferences drawn were based on the best evidence available; notably, no evidence was offered to the contrary at the time or has been offered since. In those circumstances, the psychiatrists who questioned the validity and ethics of the research undertaken took the risk of the important message that needed to be conveyed, which was that the newly adopted national immigration policy was undermining the mental health of a vulnerable minority, a conclusion that has stood the test of time. One lesson that should be learned is that individual psychiatrists would do well to consult with leaders in the field before embarking on actions of this type when issues of such profound importance in mental health are at stake.

Psychiatrists working in asylum detention centers confront a more direct ongoing ethical dilemma of attempting to serve two "masters," a well-recognized issue also known more generally as the "dual-role" dilemma (Robertson and Walter 2008). The predicament is shared to some extent with colleagues working in prisons, military installations, and institutions confining suspected terrorists (Silove et al. 2017). On the one hand, psychiatrists have a primary responsibility to act in the best interests of patients irrespective of the context; on the other hand, they are employees of a hierarchically ordered institution in which secrecy is central to the culture. The silencing of professionals reached a crisis point with the passage of legislation forbidding all personnel working in Australian detention centers from disclosing information about conditions within the institutions. The legislation was rescinded after intense pressure by representative medical associations in the country. Nevertheless, contractual arrangements with detention management companies and the strictures imposed by local authorities at Pacific Island sites continue to limit the capacity for physicians to make public their observations. For example, at the time this chapter was being written, a senior physician was expelled for allegedly taking photographs documenting an alleged human rights violation perpetrated against an inmate (Dziedzic 2018). Psychiatrists therefore continue to confront the dilemma of reconciling their ethical responsibilities in this setting. On the one hand, they have a responsibility to assist a high-risk group of asylum seekers in detention; on the other, they need to guard against the erosion of their professional independence and integrity, including their right to speak out if conditions in detention are detrimental to the mental health of their patients.

ETHICS AT THE INTERNATIONAL LEVEL: CONTROVERSIES IN GLOBAL MENTAL HEALTH

There has been a long-standing debate in the field of refugee mental health in which the cultural rights of refugees and other conflict-affected populations are seen to conflict with initiatives by Western trained psychiatrists to develop mental health services for these groups. Although appearing to be theoretical in nature, the debate has the potential to impact on real-world issues that are of key ethical importance, particularly the access that refugees have to mental health services.

Most refugees originate from culturally distinct communities that have their own traditions in identifying and responding to mental distress. At the same time, the majority of refugees reside in low- and middle-income countries in settings where conventional health services are absent or poorly developed. The question is whether two sets of rights—to preserve cultural healing practices and to provide access conventional mental health services—are incompatible. Although the debate concerning these issues originated within the refugee mental health field, it now extends to the broader domain of global mental health, a movement that aims to address the lack of core mental health services in many countries worldwide. In general, the global mental health movement has favored a utilitarian position by assuming that treatments that work in Western environments are applicable across cultures with appropriate adaptation. Global mental health therefore promotes the rollout of these approaches across low- and middle-income countries as a high priority. The model involves the transfer of skills to local health workers, who are taught to apply standardized and often manualized approaches to treating common mental health problems with the minimum of cost and technology (Patel 2012).

The contrary position, supported by proponents of what is loosely referred to as "critical psychiatry," prioritizes the protection of cultural rights, including in the domain of mental health. The overriding concern is that the imposition of Western psychiatric diagnoses and interventions on cultures where these concepts and treatments are alien undermines traditional approaches to healing that are intrinsic to the continuation of the culture. In the refugee field, the focus of criticism has been on concepts such as psychological trauma and PTSD, which are regarded as foreign to most culturally diverse societies from which the majority of refugees originate. Imposing these concepts and associated treatments on culturally diverse societies risks disrupting traditional support systems and the capacity for natural recovery from the upheavals of mass conflict and displacement.

At a more pragmatic level, there are concerns that a too rapid rollout of Western approaches to treatment may pose risks to the safety and well-being of recipient populations. In particular, for reasons of cost, first-generation psychotropic medications, which can have serious adverse effects, are often used in low- and middle-income countries. Where local workers with minimal training administer these drugs in the absence of close supervision, adverse effects are likely to be more common, resulting in potentially high levels of morbidity both in the short and longer term (Silove and Ward 2014).

Two brief vignettes drawn from the author's experience illustrate key aspects of each side of the argument.

Case 1

A team from UNSW Psychiatry with collaborators established the first emergency mental health service in Timor-Leste in the aftermath of the prolonged occupation of the country by Indonesia, an epoch that culminated in a violent upheaval in 1999 in which most community health services were destroyed. In the early period of mobilization, the team found numerous persons with severe psychosis chained to trees, locked in burnt-out basements, and incarcerated in the few prisons that were in operation. Most of these persons had received treatments by local traditional healers but with no response. In many, symptoms improved substantially after standard antipsychotic medications were administered, allowing them to be released back to their families. In one instance, a chief of a village thought to be experiencing an acute manic episode as part of a bipolar disorder had been held in leg stocks for months to prevent aggressive behavior. After a few months of treatment, he showed sufficient recovery to be able to return to his leadership role.

Case 2

Refugees fleeing persecution in West Papua, Indonesia, have resettled in the north of Australia. During a long period of engagement with the community, the UNSW Psychiatry team identified a pervasive problem of explosive anger among survivors of torture and other abuses, a pattern that led to major family and social difficulties. Some of these persons had been diagnosed with depression by doctors but antidepressant medications had proven largely ineffective in managing the angry outbursts. Qualitative research identified a culturally recognized syndrome, *Sakit Hati* (literally sick heart), which was an elaboration of a state of jealousy long recognized in civilian life in the culture but which had taken on a contemporary political meaning. Survivors of abuse tended to lapse into a state of brooding, isolation, and resentment that after a period could lead to episodes of anger and inappropriate aggression. There appeared to be no equivalent category for Sakit Hati in the western diagnostic system. On close inquiry, the underlying factor leading to the syndrome appeared to be a deep sense of helplessness that refugees felt in being unable to address the injustices of the past, to protect their families left in the homeland, and to progress the ideal of achieving national independence for their homeland. In that sense, the response pattern could only be fully understood within its cultural, historical, and political context.

These examples indicate how variations in the manifestations of mental disturbance and the context in which it occurs need to be taken into account in determining the best approach to intervention. In all settings, there is a minority of persons with severe mental illnesses who benefit from the judicious use of antipsychotic medications. In other instances, recognition of the cultural and contextual nature of a psychological reaction such as Sakit Hati is crucial to understanding the contextual meaning of the syndrome. A rigid adherence to one model (cultural or mainstream mental health) inevitably will restrict the psychiatrist in ways that are not likely to be helpful in managing the variety of presentations encountered in the refugee field.

Protagonists for a position in which cultural rights are seen as taking precedence over the need to develop conventional mental health services run the risk of denying persons with severe mental illness access to basic treatment. Those who ignore cultural issues in their haste to develop mainstream services risk undermining long-held traditions and belief systems that are intrinsic to the society. A broader ethical issue is that debates such as these, especially when polarized, can reinforce underlying prejudices, allowing donors, funders, and policy makers to continue to justify the neglect of the mentally ill. For these reasons, there is an ethical obligation for leading voices in the psychiatric profession to work towards a synthesis in which cultural rights and the right to treatment are given equal weight.

CONCLUSION

This chapter aimed to outline some of the key ethical issues encountered by psychiatrists working in the refugee field. As indicated, there are many complexities in working with refugees and at times these issues can be daunting. By adopting a multisystem approach in which a hierarchy of influences (individual, familial, community, and, related to policy making, national and international), the practitioner can achieve a comprehensive picture of the issues at stake. Ultimately, however, the clinician is faced with answering the immediate question: "What can I do to achieve the best outcome for this patient (and when relevant, his or her family and community) in this setting?" In many instances, much can be done within a one-to-one engagement in the clinical setting; in other situations, for example, in cases of intimate partner violence, the psychiatrist needs to engage the partner and other agencies to ensure the safety of all involved; and in special situations, such as when working with detained asylum seekers, the practitioner has to consider the institutional and policy framework in order to understand and respond to the situation in a fully informed manner.

An important principle in all instances is to avoid making ethical decisions in haste or in isolation. In a field in which so many factors exert an influence, no practitioner can be an expert in all the relevant areas. Refreshing one's knowledge of standing ethical guidelines and statements in psychiatry and medicine is a vital first step, followed by reference to any recent literature on the topic. Consultation with others is a critical next step. This should involve mentors and supervisors and, when possible, cultural advisors who can apprise the psychiatrist of relevant customs, beliefs, and practices in dealing with the issue within the relevant community. As indicated, there is always a need for psychiatrists to examine their own personal values and belief systems to fully understand their responses and tendencies when confronted with particularly challenging ethical issues.

For most psychiatrists, adhering to ethical principles comes naturally and forms an integral component of their practices. Placing the interests of the patient first is consistent with the humanistic mission that underpins all practice in the refugee field. The establishment of conditions of trust, compassion, and mutual respect in therapy serves both to enhance the patient's recovery process and to ensure a strong foundation in the professional relationship, making it easier to resolve any ethical issues that may arise.

KEY CLINICAL POINTS

- Maintaining confidentiality and privacy in refugee psychiatric practice is a special ethical challenge, given that interpreters are typically used and customs regarding privacy at the family level differ across cultures.

- A special issue is when the patient is found to be a perpetrator of human rights abuses. With help of colleagues, the psychiatrist may continue with treatment, but if the actions of the patient in this situation are so abhorrent that the clinician cannot continue, referral should be made elsewhere.

- Asylum seekers are increasingly stigmatized, if not outright subject to harsh punishment. Asylum seekers need clinical services and written legal reports supporting their claims. Prolonged detention, as in practice in the United States, can lead

to the perpetuation of mental health symptoms. Psychiatrists
have a responsibility to reveal human rights violations and the
effects on refugees and asylum seekers.

- Psychiatrists working in asylum detention centers confront the
  ethical dilemma of serving two "masters"—serving the best interests of the patient and yet remaining as loyal employees of
  the institution. The ethical need is to guard against the erosion
  of professional independence and integrity.

- In global mental health, there are potential ethical issues in developing conventional mental health services, which may undermine long-held traditions and belief systems intrinsic to
  the society. There is an ethical obligation for the psychiatric
  professional to work toward a synthesis in which cultural rights
  and the right to treatment are given equal weight.

- Psychiatrists need to avoid making ethical decisions in haste or
  in isolation. Consultation with knowledgeable colleagues or
  cultural advisors may be necessary.

REFERENCES

Australian Human Rights Commission: The Forgotten Children: National Inquiry Into Children in Immigration Detention 2014. Sydney, Australia,
Australian Human Rights Commission, 2014

Dziedzic S: Australia's top doctor on Nauru, Nicole Montana, arrested and deported. Australian Broadcasting Corporation, October 17, 2018. Available
at: https://www.abc.net.au/news/2018–10–17/australias-top-doctor-on-
nauru-to-be-deported-today/10385970. Accessed October 18, 2019.

Kirmayer LJ, Rousseau C, Crepeau F: Research ethics and the plight of refugees in detention. Monash Bioeth Rev 23(4):85–92, 2004 15688516

Minas IH: Detention and deception: limits of ethical acceptability in detention
research. Monash Bioeth Rev 23(4):69–77, 2004 15688513

Neuner F, Schauer M, Klaschik C, et al: A comparison of narrative exposure
therapy, supportive counseling, and psychoeducation for treating posttraumatic stress disorder in an African refugee settlement. J Consult Clin Psychol 72(4):579–587, 2004 15301642

Patel V: Global mental health: from science to action. Harv Rev Psychiatry
20(1):6–12, 2012 22335178

Rees S, Mohsin M, Tay AK, et al: Associations between bride price obligations
and women's anger, symptoms of mental distress, poverty, spouse and family conflict and preoccupations with injustice in conflict-affected Timor-
Leste. BMJ Glob Health 1(1):e000025, 2016 28588920

Rees S, Mohsin M, Tay AK, et al: Risk of perpetrating intimate partner violence amongst men exposed to torture in conflict-affected Timor-Leste. Glob Ment Health (Camb) 5:e23, 2018 29997895

Robertson MD, Walter G: Many faces of the dual-role dilemma in psychiatric ethics. Aust N Z J Psychiatry 42(3):228–235, 2008 18247198

Silove D, Ward PB: Challenges in rolling out interventions for schizophrenia. Lancet 383(9926):1362–1364, 2014 24612753

Silove D, Ventevogel P, Rees S: The contemporary refugee crisis: an overview of mental health challenges. World Psychiatry 16(2):130–139, 2017 28498581

Steel Z, Silove D: Science and the common good: indefinite, non-reviewable mandatory detention of asylum seekers and the research imperative. Monash Bioeth Rev 23(4):93–103, 2004 15688517

Steel Z, Momartin S, Bateman C, et al: Psychiatric status of asylum seeker families held for a protracted period in a remote detention centre in Australia. Aust N Z J Public Health 28(6):527–536, 2004 15707201

Steel Z, Silove D, Brooks R, et al: Impact of immigration detention and temporary protection on the mental health of refugees. Br J Psychiatry 188(1):58–64, 2006 16388071

Sultan A, O'Sullivan K: Psychological disturbances in asylum seekers held in long term detention: a participant-observer account. Med J Aust 175(11–12):593–596, 2001 11837854

Summerfield D: Afterword: against "global mental health." Transcult Psychiatry 49(3–4):519–530, 2012 23008353

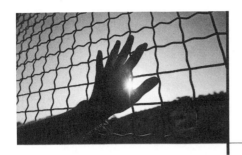

Chapter 13

OVERVIEW, PERSPECTIVES, AND RESEARCH NEEDS

George A. Keepers, M.D., FACPsych, DLFAPA

As long as humans have lived in organized groups, competed for resources, and been displaced by natural disasters, changes in climate, flood, and famine there have been refugees. Five developments distinguish the modern era from the past. First, thanks to advances in agriculture, infrastructure, and public health, modern populations are much larger than in most of human history. Second, modern warfare, despite efforts to limit incidental casualties through precision weaponry, is enormously more destructive and rapid than in the past. As the United States demonstrated in the first Iraq war, it is possible to rout and destroy large forces occupying substantial territory in a month, killing and displacing huge numbers of people. Third, although not uniformly true, the expectation of humane treatment of the displaced has been ingrained in most countries and in their political systems (Marceca et al. 2012). Fourth, the means of transportation, dramatically altered in the last century, has enabled dispersal of refugee populations to distant countries. Finally, the advent of global, instantaneous communication has created worldwide awareness of the plight of the unfortunate at an unprecedented level (Marceca 2017).

FUTURE NEEDS

What have been the consequences of these developments? The large populations that have been displaced in modern times have produced unprecedented challenges. Following World War II, the displacement of the severely traumatized European Jewish population, the establishment of Israel, and the subsequent displacement of the Palestinian population created still unresolved refugee problems. The wars in Southeast Asia created even larger populations of refugees who experienced horrific traumas. Current warfare-related refugee migrations from Middle Eastern countries into Europe and the United States have been sufficiently politically unsettling to challenge previously accepted standards of humane treatment even in the West. Ever since the Vietnam War, modern communication technology has confronted people throughout the world with the plight of traumatized civilian populations, most recently with South American groups attempting to travel to the United States to seek asylum. As previously described, the United States, European nations, and the Commonwealth nations have long been safe havens for refugees, and modern transportation technology has enabled very large groups of refugees to reach these countries. Severe trauma in these groups is very common, and the language and cultural barriers to effective treatment challenge social service and treatment programs in these countries. In the next century, climate change may severely exacerbate the problem of caring for the world's refugees. Current geographies may become uninhabitable, displacing large populations at the same time as arable land is reduced (Kummi et al. 2016). Climate refugees may well become the largest group of displaced people.

It appears likely then that immigrant and refugee populations will dramatically increase in the coming decades, a problem driven by continued conflict throughout the world and by climate change. At a policy level, countries should prepare for this impending problem. The United Nations High Commissioner for Refugees has published information that should guide member nations in establishing their policies (United Nations High Commission for Refugees 2017). The United Nations has defined a comprehensive refugee response framework and program of action. The framework, adhering to international law, establishes that individuals displaced by climate change and consequent natural disasters do fall under conventions governing the treatment of refugees. Further, individuals who do not qualify as refugees but whose countries of origin are unable to protect them against serious harm from climate change may also require international protection. The United States and other countries that are likely to become the goal of migrating populations should develop clear policies regarding this matter and should plan to invest the resources that will be needed. It is important for psychiatrists who are involved with refugee treatment programs to remain informed about these issues. Some may reasonably choose to participate in advocacy activities regarding policy issues concerning refugee protection and climate change. Studying the effectiveness of different methods coping with large dispossessed populations may enable more effective and humane resettlement, socialization, and treatment.

THE SOCIAL NEEDS OF REFUGEES

Refugees are frequently resettled in countries in which the culture, social norms, and laws are quite different from those in their country of origin. This is frequently the case for many immigrant populations in the United States, and examples abound of conflict between groups and the local community. There is much uncertainty regarding the ideal methods for integrating refugees into the host countries culture. Failure to achieve appropriate adaptation can have severe consequences for the individual refugee and it is in such a situation that the psychiatrists is likely to encounter the problem as illustrated in this case example.[1]

Case I

A Korean man in his 60s was brought to clinic by his wife with unclear complaints other than his obvious anger toward her. The couple were first-generation immigrants and had come to the United States 7 years previously. The man's spouse had been able to obtain work that supported the couple, but he was unemployed and had very limited English. He had been arrested the previous weekend after an altercation with his wife during which he struck her. She called the police, who arrested him on the basis of her report and his belligerence and inability to communicate. He spent the night in jail. He was deeply offended

---

[1]The case examples used in this chapter have been altered to remove protected health information and any personally identifiable characteristics. The cases are drawn from a cross-cultural clinic that the author conducted for a decade.

that his wife had called the police to intervene in what he regarded as a private matter. He did not understand that such actions are unlawful in the United States.

Attitudes toward domestic violence against women in many countries differ dramatically from U.S. law and custom (Oanh 2016; Trinh et al. 2016), as do attitudes toward the disciplining of children (Kim and Hong 2007). Differences in religion, legal systems, gender relations, and social custom may make adaptation to the host country very difficult for some refugees. Not enough is known about the methods and programs that attempt to improve refugee adaptation, but considerable progress has been made by studies of Australia's system (Lau et al. 2018). Rigorously conducted large studies of other systems of resettlement would be very valuable.

The Medical Needs of Refugees

In the United States refugees have been dispersed and settled throughout the country in urban, suburban, and rural settings with varying success. Psychiatrists, mental health personnel, and primary care providers may encounter these individuals in specialized programs, mental health centers, or private office and clinic practice. The medical care of these refugees is frequently compromised by barriers to treatment as illustrated by the examples below (Morris et al. 2009; Robertshaw et al. 2017).

Case 2

A 59-year-old South Korean man was referred to a psychiatric clinic specializing in the care of Korean immigrants. The clinic was staffed with a first-generation Korean immigrant psychiatric nurse practitioner who also served as translator for the psychiatrist. The patient and his wife had immigrated to the United States 12 years previously and settled in Portland. As is the case for many first-generation Korean immigrants, the patient did not speak English, attended a Korean church, and usually limited social and work activities to the Korean community. He had gone to his primary care physician multiple times with his wife as interpreter, although her English was minimal. He complained of feeling unwell, with a decline in mood, and various somatic problems (e.g., pain and weakness, particularly in his right hand). The referring physician felt that the patient's problems were psychiatric. Evaluation in the psychiatric clinic did show depression, but the patient with the aid of translation was able to express that he could not control his right hand. Examination showed clear evidence of "alien hand syndrome." An MRI demonstrated a frontal lobe glioblastoma, and he was referred to neurosurgery.

Case 3

A 50-year-old woman was advised to come to the same clinic by members of her church. She was North Korean in origin and had suffered deprivation and trauma with the imprisonment of her husband in North Korea. She escaped to South Korea and was taken in by a South Korean family. Unfortunately, she was essentially treated as an indentured worker or servant by this family. She suffered repeated beatings, including cerebral contusions. With the help of church members, she was eventually able to come to the United States and establish herself within the Korean community. Over the previous year, she and her friends had noticed declining memory, slowed thinking, and difficulties with balance. Her primary care physician was unable to address these difficulties. Evaluation in the clinic confirmed the memory problems but also elicited a history of incontinence. Examination showed poor balance and a wide-based gait. The computed tomography scan confirmed enlarged ventricles and cerebral cortex thinning. A diagnosis of hydrocephalus was made with a referral to neurosurgery.

These cases illustrate how serious medical and neurological problems of immigrants and refugees are often misdiagnosed in the primary care clinic (and no doubt in many mental health clinics). Medical screening procedures vary widely between countries, across sites within countries, and across immigration methods (Hvass and Wejse 2017). The types of conditions encountered in different immigrant, refugee, and torture victim populations vary widely, and not enough is known about this variance (Thiel de Bocanegra et al. 2018). A high index of suspicion regarding disorders that may initially present psychiatrically is important for the psychiatrist practicing in settings where these patients are encountered (Van Such et al. 2017).

TREATMENT OF PSYCHIATRIC CONDITIONS IN REFUGEES

Of course, the most common problems encountered in refugee populations are psychiatric disorders, particularly PTSD. Our understanding of the pharmacological and psychological treatment of this disorder in refugee populations is incomplete. As discussed in Chapter 5, vulnerability to the development of PTSD varies and is likely at least partially a genetic trait. This vulnerability is likely not solely linked to the serotonin transporter gene; a conserved transcriptional response to adversity (CTRA) may also be involved (Cole 2015). The CTRA response has been studied in Nepali child soldiers and found to be related to their resilience to the development of PTSD (Kohrt et al. 2017). Other candidate may emerge from genome-wide associational studies, but potential genetic diversity between refugee populations will require much work before these vulnerabilities can be reliably identified.

Although the neurocircuitry, neurochemistry, and genetics of PTSD are under active and productive investigation, clinical treatment has not yet been illuminated by all this progress. There is a substantial and promising literature directed toward the prevention of PTSD that is not relevant for the treatment of the established condition (Steckler and Risbrough 2012). The clinical guidelines in Chapter 5 for the use of prazosin are sound and based on evidence. The use of clonidine for the same purpose is based on the positive experience of patients and clinicians but the research base for this use is very limited. Comparisons of the two agents are lacking, and other α-adrenergic antagonists might also be effective. Developing the evidence base for pharmacological intervention in the nightmares, enhanced startle response, and irritability associated with PTSD would be a valuable addition to the clinical knowledge base.

Similarly, the use of selective serotonin reuptake inhibitors (SSRIs) in PTSD, particularly sertraline and paroxetine, is supported by evidence, but there is little reason to think that other SSRIs would not also be effective. Clinicians have noted some advantages to using tricyclic antidepressants, but these agents have not been systematically studied for this purpose. Genetic and cultural factors complicate pharmacological studies in these populations. There is no guarantee that an agent that provides relief in Vietnamese patients will work for Syrian refugees. Nonetheless, systematic, placebo-controlled, or active-drug comparisons would be helpful in establishing the utility of tricyclics for PTSD.

A variety of intriguing methods for treatment of PTSD have been proposed, often combining psychotherapy and a pharmacological or brain stimulation method. For example, a study of repetitive transcranial magnetic stimulation used to augment cognitive processing therapy in veterans showed earlier PTSD symptom reduction that was sustained for 6 months (Kozel et al. 2018). Other methods, including deep brain stimulation, are being considered for testing. However, the completed and proposed studies are in patients from Western, industrialized, rich, and democratic nations, and the treatments may not be effective when applied to patients from different cultures and genetic backgrounds.

A similar conundrum applies to the psychotherapeutic treatment of PTSD in refugees. There is a strong evidence base for treatment of PTSD with prolonged exposure therapy, cognitive processing therapy, and trauma-focused cognitive-behavioral therapy (Watkins et al. 2018). However, the clinical experiences described in this book indicate that these methods are not helpful with severely traumatized patients from other cultures. In fact, the evidence base for the effectiveness of these methods consists entirely of studies conducted on patients from Western, educated, industrialized, rich, and developed nations. A Cochrane review of evidence for the effectiveness of multiple psychotherapeutic methods, including the ones mentioned above, in torture victims found very few methodologically sound studies, no immediate improvement in PTSD symptoms, and minimal improvement in a few patients at 6 months (Patel et al. 2016). The study raised ethical concerns regarding the use of prolonged exposure and trauma-focused methods in these patients because evidence of worsening symptoms was found in many of the patients (Patel et al. 2016).

Refugees also suffer from other familiar psychiatric conditions that psychiatrists routinely treat. Psychiatrists will generally be quite comfortable in addressing these clinical situations. Sometimes, however, these conditions may present in unusual ways because of language and cultural issues that alter their presentation as illustrated by the case below.

Case 4

A first-generation immigrant in her 70s was brought to clinic by a concerned daughter. She had been diagnosed for many years with a severe anxiety disorder and was seeking a doctor to prescribe the clonazepam that she had been taking. Her presentation at the clinic was alarming. Her speech was slurred, she stumbled and nearly fell several times, and she had many bruises on her arms and legs from previous falls. She revealed that she had been taking clonazepam 10 mg daily for several years. A prolonged process of relationship establishment and treatment negotiation made it possible to gradually reduce the dose over the subsequent 8 months. When the dosage of her clonazepam reached 2 mg/day, paranoid thinking and delusional material emerged, and it became apparent that she had an underlying psychosis. Her symptoms responded well to a low dose of olanzapine.

At other times the clinical circumstances will be entirely routine and successful treatment will be enabled with appropriate attention to correct diagnosis, appropriate psychopharmacological treatment, and attention to compliance. Patients may have difficulty communicating the reasons for noncompliance. A careful investigation of therapeutic effect and adverse reactions will usually guide the clinician toward a successful treatment as happened in this final case.

Case 5

A young mother, a Korean immigrant who worked supporting her family, developed schizophrenia. She was hospitalized several times and was eventually referred to clinic. She had been treated with several antipsychotics but had discontinued them shortly after each hospitalization. With the help of an interpreter, we learned the reasons that had led to this pattern. Haloperidol made her feel very restless. On olanzapine, she slept all the time and gained weight. Lithium caused severe tremor that she could not tolerate. She was, understandably, reluctant to take medications, and her insight into her illness was limited. With appropriate counseling, reassurance, and frequent visits, she agreed to further medication treatment. The first trial of risperidone failed because of parkinsonian side effects, but the second treatment tried was aripiprazole. She responded extremely well to 5 mg/day and was able to resume work and take care of her children effectively.

FINAL REFLECTIONS

The need for refuge for the dispossessed has never been greater than at the present time, and it is likely that this need will only become larger in the future. The medical and psychiatric treatment of refugees is an essential but insufficient response to this crisis. Nations with the means must be willing to invest in the fostering of unfortunate peoples displaced from their homes by war, oppression, famine, and the ravages of human-caused climate change. Humane procedures for entry and resettlement, provision of social services, and innovative methods of integration and adaptation will be necessary. Kindness, tolerance, and the desire to help those in need in our communities are essential to success. In the shadow of the end of World War II, the nations of the globe agreed to these principles in 1951. Those agreements have endured for decades and must not be abandoned now.

In this volume we have outlined how our colleagues can contribute to this effort. It begins with our willingness to help those in need no matter how difficult the task. And the task is difficult. Providing care to the victims of the world's sorrows is technically difficult. Language, culture, differences in social expectations, and our limited knowledge in how to help are all barriers to success. But even more difficult is to hear, understand, and empathize with those who have suffered so much. Tears are inevitable in even reading of these tragic stories. Yet the work also gives meaning and joy. Our nation has always welcomed the dispossessed. We should do no less.

> Give me your tired, your poor, your huddled masses
> yearning to breathe free. The wretched refuse of
> your teeming shore. Send these, the homeless, the
> tempest-tost to me. I lift my lamp beside the golden
> door.
>
> Emma Lazarus

KEY CLINICAL POINTS

- Increasing numbers of refugees resettled in many communities in the United States are likely in the coming decades.

- Different cultural and social expectations, coupled with barriers to communication, may result in adverse outcomes for patients resettled in the United States.

- Psychiatrists should maintain a high level of clinical alertness to the presence of medical and neurological conditions that can mimic psychiatric disorders. Refugees, depending on origin, may suffer from unusual (in the United States) parasitic, infectious, and other diseases.

- PTSD in refugees and victims of torture requires different approaches to treatment than PTSD related to combat or civilian trauma in patients in the United States.

- Psychiatrists should feel confident that they can treat many common psychiatric disorders in refugees and that they will be providing much needed help to the dispossessed.

REFERENCES

Cole SW: Human social genomics. PLoS Genet 10(8):e1004601, 2015 25166010

Hvass AM, Wejse C: Systematic health screening of refugees after resettlement in recipient countries: a scoping review. Ann Hum Biol 44(5):475–483, 2017 28562071

Kim E, Hong S: First generation Korean American parents' perceptions of discipline. J Prof Nurs 23(1):60–68, 2007 17292135

Kohrt BA, Wothman CM, Adhikari RP, et al: Psychological resilience and the gene regulatory impact of post traumatic stress in Nepali child soldiers. Proc Natl Acad Sci U S A 113(29):8156–8161, 2017 27402736

Kozel FA, Motes MA, Didehbani N, et al: Repetitive TMS to augment cognitive processing therapy in combat veterans of recent conflicts with PTSD: a randomized clinical trial. J Affect Disord 229:506–514, 2018 29351885

Kummi M, de Moel H, Salvucci G, et al: Over the hills and further away from the coast: geospatial patterns of human and environment over the 20th to the 21st century. Environmental Research Letters 11(3):1–15, 2016

Lau W, Silove D, Edwards B, et al: Adjustment of refugee children and adolescents in Australia: outcomes from wave three of the Building a New Life in Australia study. BMC Med 16(1):157, 2018 30176864

Marceca M: Migration and health from a public health perspective, in People's Movements in the 21st Century: Risks, Challenges, and Benefits. Edited by Muenstermann I, Rijeka, Croatia, IntechOpen, 2017, pp 103–127

Marceca M, Geraci S, Baglio G, et al: Immigrants health protection: political, institutional and social perspectives at international and Italian level. Italian Journal of Public Health 9:2427–7498, 2012

Morris MD, Popper ST, Rodwell TC, et al: Healthcare barriers of refugees post-resettlement. J Community Health 34(6):529–538, 2009 19705264

Patel N, C de C Williams A, Kellezi B: Reviewing outcomes of psychological interventions with torture survivors: conceptual, methodological and ethical Issues. Torture 26(1):2–16, 2016 27857002

Robertshaw L, Dhesi S, Jines LL: Challenges and facilitators for health professionals providing primary healthcare for refugees and asylum seekers in high-income countries: a systematic review and thematic synthesis of qualitative research. BMJ Open 7(8):e015981, 2017 27857002

Steckler T, Risbrough V: Pharmacological treatment of PTSD—established and new approaches. Neuropharmacology 62(2):617–627, 2012 21736888

Thiel de Bocanegra H, Carter-Pokras O, Ingleby JD, et al: Addressing refugee health through evidence-based policies: a case study. Ann Epidemiol 28(6):411–419, 2018 28554498

Trinh OT, Oh J, Choi S, et al: Changes and socioeconomic factors associated with attitudes towards domestic violence among Vietnamese women aged 15–49: findings from the Multiple Indicator Cluster Surveys, 2006–2011. Glob Health Action 9:29577, 2016 26950567

United Nations High Commission for Refugees: Climate change, disaster, and displacement in the Global Compacts: UNHCR's perspectives. November 2017. Available at: https://www.unhcr.org/en-us/5a12f9577.pdf. Accessed October 21, 2019.

Van Such M, Lohr R, Beckman T, et al: Extent of diagnostic agreement among medical referrals. J Eval Clin Pract 23(4):870–874, 2017 28374457

Watkins LE, Sprang KR, Rothbaum BO: Treating PTSD: a review of evidence-based psychotherapy interventions. Front Behav Neurosci 12:258, 2018 30450043

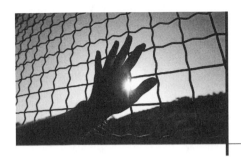

POSTSCRIPT

J. David Kinzie, M.D., FACPsych, DLFAPA
George A. Keepers, M.D., FACPsych, DLFAPA

We along with most of the other authors in this book have spent an important portion of our professional lives treating immigrants and refugees. We have come to know many of them very well. Whether from Asia, Africa, the Middle East, Europe, or Central America, their stories have familiar themes. Refugees come to the United States to escape wars, genocide, lawlessness, random murders, starvation, extreme cruelty, and torture. Most have lost family members to ethnic cleansing, massacres, forced starvation, extrajudicial killing, and desperate attempts to flee. They come, sometimes with children, without their previous society or friends to a new place, with little or no knowledge of our culture or the ability to speak our dominant language, afraid and often alone.

We have listened to their stories, which, providing much more than a clinical interview, tell of their attempts to survive, now familiar to us, while war gangs, or even local police authorities in their midst, intimidated and killed their family members.

We have learned about their heroic escapes from their homes to refugee camps, where there was starvation and limited safety. Even in United Nations–sponsored refugee camps, there were rapes, theft of what little food or belongings they had, deaths from poor or no medical care, and little hope things could improve. Some lucky ones got picked by lottery to come to the United States, while others came on their own, asking for asylum from a likely death if they returned to their home country.

The refugees had many symptoms, with those of PTSD and depression being most common, but symptoms of psychosis and traumatic brain injury were also prevalent. Hypertension and diabetes were very common. And, in addition, there was the adjustment to a new culture and a new country. And, especially for asylum seekers, there was the constant fear of being deported.

As our treatment relationship continued, the relationships among the doctor, counselor, and patient grew as we communicated deeply about human misery and the most basic examples of human loss. The refugees were desperately fighting not just for their lives but for the totality of their own human existence, as well as for the existence of everything they had ever known. Because almost all of what the refugees had valued and known and cherished had been brutally and violently snatched away, the relationship to our clinic became very important to them.

We as doctors began to celebrate with them the joys in their achieving asylum, becoming U.S. citizens, and the everyday successes of their children, such as going to school, marriages, and births of children and grandchildren. We grieved with them over deaths in their community or family, over the struggles they had raising children in this new culture, over the problems they had finding work and housing, and sometimes over their own or a family member's diagnosis of severe medical illness. Sometimes, they were also coming to terms with and accepting their own or a family member's diagnosis of mental illness.

In the therapy groups, there were times of celebrations with staff and volunteers, such as Tet (Vietnamese New Year), Eid al-Fitr after Ramadan, and Cinco de Mayo. And, in turn, the refugees joined in American celebrations of Thanksgiving and Christmas.

We, doctors and patients, enriched each other's lives, and we admired the patients' resilience and lack of anger or hostility. As the refugees moved into the mainstream of American life, acquiring skills that enhanced their own American economic life, they seemed as if they were over their past traumas. They were not. Some still suffer from insecurity, fear, and nightmares. They remain vulnerable to threats.

We who work with and feel privileged to know refugees understand well how much their diversity adds to and enriches American culture, and yet?

And yet, at this point in our history, there are Americans who say they hate immigrants and refugees. We see it in current writings and speeches as refugees are referred to as animals or vermin, as infestations, as aliens, or as "an invasion." Increasingly vocal white nationalists appear to see refugees as a stain on our country, a takeover of a mythical white country. The hatred is directed toward blacks, Africans, Asians, Hispanics, Muslims, Jews, and even LGBTQ communities. The hatred arises out of fear of losing the "whiteness" of American life. This hatred leads to discrimination, angry threats, and hostile jokes, but also to violence, such as the dramatic experiences in Charlottesville, Pittsburgh, and El Paso have shown.

The refugees see this also, and their fear now is much more evident. Refugee women, especially those with hijabs, are afraid of going out alone. Some refugees are afraid of enduring insults, angry stares, or even violence. The safety they sought in America seems less secure and more unpredictable now without even the U.S. government to protect them.

After the Muslim ban was put in place in 2017, a newly arrived Somali refugee was asked by her young daughter, "Mommy, where can we go now?"

The refugees have our sympathies, but "sympathy," as Susan Sontag has written, "is a fragile emotion." It must constantly be renewed against ongoing public hatred. Sympathy can wither without support from friends or the community.

Hatred also is a fragile emotion. It must be supported by others who continually talk of the threat and danger of "the others" coming here to America. It is necessary to stoke fears to keep hate going.

Maybe . . . just maybe, if some white nationalists were to meet some refugees, and they were able to listen to each other, each group could see and begin to understand the other group's desire for a better life for their children, experience a peace within themselves and others, and even experience joy in learning about other's ways of living and thinking.

Then, the hatred might wither and die.

Index

Page numbers printed in **boldface** type refer to tables or figures.